SHAPING THE
Motherhood
OF INDIGENOUS MEXICO

Vania Smith-Oka

Vanc

© 2013 by Vanderbilt University Press
Nashville, Tennessee 37235
All rights reserved
First printing 2013

This book is printed on acid-free paper.
Manufactured in the United States of America

Library of Congress Cataloging-in-Publication Data on file

LC control number 2012036591
LC classification number F1219.3.W6S65 2012
Dewey class number 972'.49—dc23

ISBN 978-0-8265-1917-7 (cloth)
ISBN 978-0-8265-1918-4 (paperback)
ISBN 978-0-8265-1919-1 (e-book)

SHAPING THE
Motherhood
OF INDIGENOUS
MEXICO

*For Dolly, who sat on my lap when I began,
and for Kalpana, who nursed while I finished.*

Contents

Acknowledgments

THIS STUDY EMERGES FROM THE LIVES OF THE WOMEN OF AMATLÁN. First and foremost are the women who participated and who shared their stories, concerns, joys, and fears. It is thanks to their boundless generosity in sharing their sorrows and laughter that this book was even possible. While all the wonderful people I met in Amatlán will remain anonymous, I hope that their voices come through in this narrative. I am particularly grateful for the open-armed hospitality of everyone in the village. They invited me into their homes and told their stories about their lives and experiences without hesitation. I have been fortunate to make their friendships. Additionally, the support and good humor of the teachers and clinicians was integral in understanding the larger context for education and health relevant to these women's lives.

Funding for this book came from various sources over the years: the Provost Award of the University of Illinois at Chicago, the Foundation for the Advancement of Mesoamerican Studies, and the Kellogg Institute for International Studies at the University of Notre Dame. The Institute for Scholarship in the Liberal Arts, College of Arts and Letters, University of Notre Dame, funded parts of my data collection and also provided a generous book subvention. Notable people at Notre Dame supported this intellectual endeavor, particularly Holly Rivers, Sharon Schierling, Ted Beatty, Laurie Arnold, Patricia Base, Agustín Fuentes, and Tom Merluzzi.

In Mexico, support came from institutions such as the Centro de Investigaciones y Estudios Superiores en Antropología Social (CIESAS), the Secretaría de Desarrollo Social (SEDESOL), and the Consejo Nacional de Población (CONAPO). Dr. Jesús Ruvalcaba Mercado and Dr.

Juan Manuel Pérez Zevallos from CIESAS guided me in navigating the world of Mexican anthropology and the Huasteca region. Their generous invitations to present my work at their conferences and publications have been extraordinary. Various directors at SEDESOL (particularly Dr. Gustavo Merino) and CONAPO aided in understanding the bureaucracies of Mexican development ministries. I am grateful to the political authorities of Ixhuatlán de Madero for allowing this work to take place; Ana Lilia Castro was especially kind, taking me under her wing and helping to smooth my entrance into the area.

A great many people at the University of Illinois at Chicago and the Field Museum of Natural History were integral in shaping me intellectually as an anthropologist: Anna Roosevelt, John Monaghan, Brian Bauer, Joel Palka, Gayatri Reddy, Mark Liechty, Chapurukha Kusimba, Sylvia Vatuk, and Lawrence Keeley. Marisa Fontana, Andreas Dahl-Hansen, Mark Golitko, Emilie Utigard, Jeff Buechler, Shannon Freeman, Rebecca Osborne, and Lisa Niziolek provided entertaining and much-needed breaks from what was oftentimes the onerous task of writing.

I am especially indebted to Alan and Pamela Sandstrom, from Indiana University–Purdue University Fort Wayne, who allowed me to continue their intellectual and personal legacy in Amatlán. For this, I am eternally grateful.

I owe a special thanks to my friends and colleagues in the Department of Anthropology at the University of Notre Dame. Most significant among these have been Jim McKenna, Mark Schurr, Agustín Fuentes, Deb Rotman, Diane Pribbernow, Angie Schumacher, Joanne Mack, and Patrick Gaffney. Ian Kuijt and Meredith Chesson warmed my insides with good food and stories, while also igniting the fire under me to complete this book. Many others fortified me with emotional support, lighting the way with friendship and laughter: Donna Glowacki, Larissa Fast, Danielle Joyner, Deborah Shamoon, Jessica Collett, Omar Lizardo, Daniel Lende, Devi Snively, Neil MacDonald, Eric Lindland, and Machelle Lee. I am most especially thankful to Carolyn Nordstrom, whose enthusiasm for my work helped to untangle many of the intellectual cobwebs along the way.

My greatest intellectual debt is owed to Cynthia Mahmood, Susan Blum, and Chapurukha Kusimba for their careful reading of various drafts of the manuscript and for their invaluable comments and advice to a neophyte book writer. It was thanks to the Notre Dame anthropology department's writing club, spearheaded and managed with razor-sharp wit by Sue Sheridan, that this work took its first steps into the light. My cowriters in crime, Jada Benn-Torres, Donna Glowacki, Gabriel Torres, Catherine Bolten, and Rahul Oka, provided the structure I needed to complete this book.

Many colleagues across the discipline contributed to the intellectual process of this book: Lauren Fordyce, Crystal Patil, Alyson Young, Lara Braff, Carole Browner, Lynn Morgan, Carolyn Smith-Morris, and Aminata Maraesa. I am especially grateful to Margaret MacDonald, who told me just how great an experience publishing with Vanderbilt University Press would be.

It has been thanks to the unwavering support of Michael Ames, director of Vanderbilt University Press, that this book is finally seeing the light. He waited patiently for chapters to trickle in and performed near-miracles in helping to transform a solid idea into a great book. The staff at Vanderbilt was always gracious and supportive. I am especially thankful to Sue Havlish and Joell Smith-Borne for moving the project into its final stages, as well as to Kathleen Kageff for excellent copyediting support and suggestions. The anonymous reviewers provided important insights into the nature of development, medical anthropology, and reproduction that helped to guide this book into its current form.

Judy Torgus, my copy editor and friend, gave me several gentle pushes to put hands to keyboard when much of this book was still in my head. I am very grateful to Stephanie Fairhurst, who joined my fieldwork in Amatlán one summer. Her enthusiasm and joy of discovery was contagious. She generously allowed one of her photos to be used in this book. Important help with references and note transcription was provided by several students at Notre Dame, notably Carolina Goncalves, Kirsten Prabhudas, Jill Schroeder, Hallie Brewster, Crystal Truong, and Cara Davies. Chelsea Gans from Lawrence University provided superb last minute help when needed. Special thanks goes to my student assistant, Caitlin Monesmith, whose enthusiasm for vectors, Photoshop, and maps transformed this book.

My army of babysitters—Emily Lambert, Shelly Birch, Christine Dombroski, Katie Melloh, Callie Merriam, Kelly Colas, Alyssa Hummel, Anna Fish, and Elizabeth Andrews—in whose capable arms my daughter found beloved alloparenting, allowed me several weekly hours to feverishly write. I particularly wish to thank Julie McCaw, on whose judgment and kindness I grew to rely, and whose mothering was so often indistinguishable from my own.

My Indian family was supportive throughout this process. Lali Oka's haikus brought smiles during dark times, and Kaka and Maushi Joshi lovingly gave emotional and spiritual support and allowed me to trust that dawn does eventually come after the night. My late parents-in-law, Chandrashekhar and Kalpana Oka, did not live to see the completion of this dream, but their love was still felt.

My loving thanks goes to my family. My siblings Odette Smith and Jerome Smith lent sympathetic ears over the years and patiently understood my feverish writing during family reunions. My sister Natalia Smith and her husband, Jonathan Rivers, in discussions that were much needed and often heated, provided public health perspectives that I hope I have done justice to here. My parents, Christopher and Pauline Smith, helped in all capacities, from acting as cheerleaders and babysitters to serving as intellectual sounding boards. Their careful reviews of various drafts went over and above parental duty and helped to transform the manuscript into its final form. I am indebted to them in more ways than I can possibly express.

The deepest feelings of gratitude and love go to my husband, Rahul Oka, and to our beautiful daughter, Kalpana. Each, in different ways, has been a midwife to this book. The midnight discussions about development, indigeneity, and reproduction were the intellectual cauldrons within which so many of the ideas in this book simmered. My own transformation into a mother to Kalpana gave me an insider's glimpse into the maelstrom of feelings and concerns experienced by mothers across the globe. This change, in turn, became my strength and allowed me to write this book.

Acronyms and Agencies

CDI: Comisión Nacional para el Desarrollo de los Pueblos Indígenas; National Commission for the Development of Indigenous Peoples

CONAPO: Consejo Nacional de Población; National Population Council of Mexico

ICPD: International Conference on Population and Development

Oportunidades: Literally "Opportunities"; the state-run conditional cash transfer program that seeks to alleviate extreme poverty

PAN: Partido Acción Nacional; National Action Party

PRI: Partido Revolucionario Institucional; Institutional Revolutionary Party

PRD: Partido de la Revolución Democrática; Democratic Revolutionary Party

Procampo: Pro-farm; a state-administered subsidy for farmers

Progresa: Former name of Oportunidades

SEDESOL: Secretaría de Desarrollo Social; Ministry of Social Development

A Word on Nahuatl Pronunciation

THE NAHUATL ALPHABET WAS ADAPTED FROM THE SPANISH ALPHABET after colonial contact, and thus it borrowed most of its letters from Spanish.[1] Convention has changed over the past couple of decades to incorporate more phonetic spelling by including K instead of a hard C, S instead of a soft C, W instead of U followed by a vowel, and so on. The letters CH, M, N, P, T, and Y are pronounced in Nahuatl as they are in English.

Stress in Nahuatl is primarily in the second to last syllable unless otherwise indicated with an accent. So it is AmaTLÁN but TonanTZINtla.

Below I have included various forms of pronunciation that might be needed by a reader of this book.

C   Can either be a soft C (pronounced as an S) if before E or I, or a hard C (pronounced as a K) if before an A, O, or U.

CU   Pronounced as KW, as in "quick."

H   On its own, not in conjunction with CH, UH, or HU, it often represents a glottal stop.

HU   Pronounced as W.

J   Pronounced as H, as in "house."

K   Always a hard C.

LL   It is a long L rather than a palatal L, as it is in Spanish.

TL   This is a lateral fricative and is pronounced as a single sound released on either side of the tongue.

TS or
TZ   The T is voiced, and the sound is simultaneously T and S, not one followed by the other.

U   If followed by a vowel it is pronounced as W. A silent H can appear before a U when it begins a syllable or when it is between vowels.

X   Pronounced as SH, as in "shell."

A, E, I,
and O   The vowels. Pronounced as in Spanish.

Introduction

Burst Uterus and Spoiled Milk

THE PICKUP TRUCK BOUNCED ALONG THE RUTTED ROAD. TITO WAS GIG-gling in the backseat, enchanted by the constant honking of the passing trucks loaded down by their enormous cargos of oranges bound for the cities. His grandmother Esperanza sat composedly on the seat beside him, looking out at the rapidly passing scenery outside her open window. Occasionally she would shush Tito's exclamations impatiently. The hot June morning sun had melted the tarmac in places, creating black waves of lava-looking material. Sweat poured down my back, gluing me to the vinyl seat. We headed down the two-lane road toward Alamo, where we would intersect with the Pan-American Highway. We were on our way to the Poza Rica airport to pick up a student guest.

What was curious about this trip was that the farther away we got from the indigenous village of Amatlán, the farther away we got from *México profundo*—from deep and profound Mexico.[1] Simultaneously, we also got closer to mainstream Mexican culture, to the *México imaginario*.[2] I was particularly struck by how issues of place and belonging were suddenly reversed. In Amatlán, I was the neophyte and the one who knew nothing, and everyone else was an expert. But the further we traveled away from the village, the more my "knowledge" of the world we were entering grew—from road signs, to air-conditioned convenience stores, to parking lots—until I was the "authority." Custom in Amatlán dictated that Esperanza, as my host and an older member of the society, be in charge of my life in the village—advising me on whom to speak with, where to go, and how to be careful in dangerous situations. But now in "my world" I was no longer allowed to defer decisions to Esperanza but was expected to be in charge of the whole expedition. This collision of two ways of life spoke volumes about the daily struggle of the Amatlán villagers to make sense of their rapidly changing world. Questions about place and belonging, about insider and outsider, and about the externalities of our interactions ran through my mind.

On this morning, as the Postectli hill glistened far away in the haze,[3] we passed the many small villages dotting the road; thatch-roofed mud houses coexisted with concrete homes, brightly painted and with wrought-iron gates. Small clinics with health slogans painted on them, extolling the virtues of vaccination and prenatal care, stood next to primary schools and *telebachilleratos*.[4] Proud, gleaming *galeras* stood in villages that could afford them.[5] The smell of the smoke from the cooking fires was indistinguishable from the smell of the smoke of burning fields being prepared for the approaching wet season. Chickens scurried across the road at inopportune moments, yet they always seemed to make it to safety. Women and men stood under the shade of trees, waiting for the ramshackle local buses to make an appearance and take them to their destination. The older women wore indigenous clothes and a folded towel on their braided heads to protect themselves from the brutal sun. Younger women, while wearing the ubiquitous towel, were dressed in polyester and viscose dresses and had gelled their hair into tight ponytails. Men rarely wear indigenous clothes, unless they are elderly; most of them were dressed in dark polyester trousers and button-down cotton shirts. All carried a *morral*—a woven straw bag—over their shoulders. We could see many people toiling at their agricultural or domestic labor—men walking along the road laden with a sack of dried corn, women carrying heavy loads of wood to cook their family's meals, or women washing clothes in the small, cloudy streams, plumes from their detergent swirling in the slow water.

Once we reached the highway our speed decreased to a crawl as the road was congested with buses and orange-laden trucks all trying to scramble past the newly built tollbooth. Two hours after leaving Amatlán we reached the almost invisible turn-off to the Poza Rica airport, passing a military checkpoint with lazing staff. Leaving the pickup truck crookedly parked in the middle of the empty parking lot, we walked into the small air-conditioned airport building. This region is heavily dependent on the petroleum business, and the airport reflected this: though most people in the building were suit-wearing and briefcase-carrying men, the industrial smell of Poza Rica insinuated itself into every corner. Our little group attracted a lot of stares.

Oblivious to the stares, Esperanza and Tito looked fixedly at the airplanes parked on the tarmac. A small plane was parked just outside the window, and we gravitated toward it. Esperanza remarked as we waited, "They are very big! Why then when they fly overhead do they look so small?" Before I could wrap my mind around the physics in the answer, they announced the arrival of the plane carrying Stephanie, our guest student. She was easy to pick out from the small group of travelers, and after warm greetings were exchanged, we headed out to the truck to return home.

The sequence of events, and the sequence of my emotions and thoughts about place and space, occurred in reverse. I was once again the stranger and outsider, and as the kilometers brought us closer to Amatlán, Esperanza became the expert once more. She had the experiential knowledge about how many turkeys were needed to make a *zacahuil*, how to choose the most tender corn to make *xamitl* for her family, how to bathe newborn babies to lessen the heat of the birth blood, and how to manage her family's small income garnered from farming and from government cash grants.[6] An exemplary mother by village standards, Esperanza struggled, along with most other indigenous women in the region, under the classification of "bad mother." This classification marked the relationship that women like Esperanza had with welfare and health-care institutions, shaping their interaction with mainstream Mexico.

Shaping Motherhood

Mainstream Mexican views of indigenous women center on them as problematic mothers, and development programs have been created with the goals of, among many other things, helping these women become "good mothers." Economic incentives and conditional cash transfers are the vehicles for achieving this goal. Such programs emerge from middle-class perceptions of comfort and stability: if one has a certain income or amount of money, then naturally certain other behaviors will follow to benefit the individual but, most importantly, to benefit society in some way. As Stacy Pigg (1997:233) shows in her work among birth attendants in Nepal, development programs dismantle "different sociocultural realities" while simultaneously taking them into account. In the process, however, they create generic models that rarely can be mapped from one culture onto another (Ginsburg and Rapp 1995).

What has been created in the welfare programs of Mexico is a *social* structural adjustment program where the women receiving the money must make changes to their lives in order to continue receiving the money. Their practices within the domestic sphere are to be modified and rationalized (Vaughn 2000) to match those of the mainstream. The rationalizing and self-care directives of the modernization of Mexico refashion ideas from the Enlightenment, where science is of great importance and where human consciousness can be emancipated from an immature state of ignorance and error—a state of being that requires the guidance from someone in authority in order to function properly.[8] Some would call these cash incentives a type of bribe, which has the goal of socially engineering women into a vision of normalized and normative motherhood. Ultimately, because the conditional cash transfer program has been provided to all indigenous women in the country, the monetary incentives have the unintended consequence of erasing the women's indigeneity by purposefully replacing indigenous forms of mothering with mainstream and *mestizo* forms.[7] Women are expected to follow orders and change their ways, with the expected outcome that they will then have a fuller and more complete life. If any woman opposes these directives, she is called a bad mother.

Within these Mexican programs, concern frequently centers on family planning and the number of children a woman has. One clinician stated,

> I explain to the women who already have two [or] three children that they should get an operation. I explain it to them using a balloon. I tell them that when you inflate it the first time it grows and looks pretty, and when it deflates it is all right except for being a little bit baggy. But I show them that by the fourth or fifth time it is inflated it bursts. Although the uterus does not actually burst, each time it becomes bigger and baggier and it will detach [from its place]. This is because they do not let it rest; they are constantly using it.

The image of a ballooning uterus is a wonderful symbol of the "excessive fertility" embodied by indigenous women. The woman in such an image seems almost to become a passive participant between a penis and her uterus, the latter of which is "filled" at certain intervals almost without the woman's having any say in the matter. This balloon image confronts the joys and risks of motherhood, by showing how women's alienation from their bodies results in passivity. Women's passivity has been considered one of the primary culprits in Mexico's population and reproductive trajectory. Various twentieth-century population campaigns were thus aimed at producing only willed and desired pregnancies.[8] Laveaga states, "If everyone was to live better [then] people needed to become more active as citizens and take control of their reproductive decisions" (2007:25).

Not only were children supposed to be "chosen," but also, symbolically, motherhood is supposed to be about what a mother can provide for her children. Biologically, this would be the production of breast milk. Fátima, the mother of three children, explained that she breastfed her children "because formula costs money. . . . They need to be fed so they don't suffer." Breastfeeding is seen as a good thing, as something a good mother does. Women breastfeed to "indulge and nurture" their children, as one of the women told me. A good mother nurtures and nurses her child and gives it all the love and nutrients it needs for life.

But the boundary between good and bad mothering can be very thin. A woman can suddenly become a "bad mother" if she willfully continues to feed her children "not good enough" milk. Indigenous women are told that their own bodies are failing them and that what they produce is not good enough for children to consume. Fátima's words encapsulate this sentiment: "The doctor says we should take [the breast] away at four or five months. That it is no longer good. [He says] that 'instead of feeding [the child], you deprive it.'" Such words condemn the very person of these women. They are seen as failures to themselves and to their children, and even to the state. Their own bodies cannot feed their children; they are unable to provide them the means to grow into healthy adults. Consequently, any mother who continues to feed her child breast milk is seen as harming that child and not allowing it to develop properly. Mothers across the village have found themselves having to nurse in secret, assuring the physicians and nurses that they have weaned their children of the ostensibly watery and nutrition-poor liquid.

The ideas of a baggy, overused womb and of watery milk provide powerful images that encapsulate many of the naturalizing and binary ideas existent in Mexico regarding indigenous motherhood. Indigenous motherhood is considered problematic in many ways. Present within Mexico are larger institutions of modernity—such as social welfare and economic incentive programs—that shape marginalized and indigenous women's motherhood. A set of binary categories provides the basic structure for socially adjusting women's motherhood. With categories for mothers—such as compliant/noncompliant, good/bad, Mexican/indigenous, and responsible/irresponsible—exist quick labels that carry deep, historical, and cultural meanings and inequities, with very real social, political, and economic implications for the women themselves.

Motherhood, and the products made by mothers—whether of their own body or their own actions—must therefore be controlled and modified into the mainstream. The mother's products, and her mothering actions, must be replaced by the correct forms encouraged—and developed—by the state. And in the same way that the indigenousness of the women must be made *mestizo* and mainstream, so too must their bodies and motherhood. These "eugenic controls" (Ginsburg and Rapp 1991:314) of the women's individual and social bodies aim to refashion them into good producers of good citizens. At this point, the Mexican state can, through its cash transfer and welfare programs, step in with its nutritional supplements, in effect making the women and their bodies obsolete. And more insidiously, any woman who goes against these directives can simply be classified as a bad mother—a moniker that carries with it significant consequences.

Stumbling onto Motherhood

When I first drove into Amatlán in January 2004, my plan was to re-search the changing role of healing specialists. I arrived armed with piles of old newspapers to dry what I, perhaps romantically, imagined would be hundreds of medicinal plants I would collect from the knowledgeable specialists as we walked around the forest. I hoped to focus on the ways that their healing practices and access to medicinal plants affected the forest landscape. But I arrived at a crucial time for the village, a time when the slow accumulation of change from the economic programs had created a tipping point in the people's medical sphere. Religious conversion through Pentecostal faiths had arrived twenty years previously, which had irrevocably changed the religious landscape (Sandstrom 1991).[9] An increase in migration from the rural areas to cities had affected the flow of money and goods in the village. The introduction of a medical clinic in the neighboring village of Tepatepec had changed the health beliefs and practices of the people. And the enrollment of a large proportion of women in Oportunidades had affected the women's interaction with the world outside the village. There was also no forest to speak of. No longer were people directly dependent on medicinal plants and healing specialists for their health needs, but neither were they fully accustomed to receiving medical care from biomedicine. Their health care existed in a kind of limbo, where unease and suspicion about both types of medical care were present for many of the people.

My own exploration into motherhood, and into the motherhood of my friends in Amatlán, was a circuitous but ultimately extremely rewarding process. Faced with a research project disappearing before my eyes, I began to do what every good field researcher does: talk to people. During this "ethnographically observed practice" (Goldstein 2003:44), I found my attention taken up by the medical concerns of the women in the village, who spoke about forced sterilizations, about the curtailing of their motherhood, and of the modification of their mothering. What emerged from these intimate conversations was a fascinating portrayal of indigenous motherhood and the state structures intent on its change.

My entrance into Amatlán was facilitated by Alan Sandstrom, who had carried out in-depth research there for over three decades.[10] In 2002, he invited me to accompany him and his wife, Pamela, to visit the village as a side trip to a conference we were attending in the region. As my enthusiasm and enchantment with the village was evident after the visit, Alan told me I was welcome to carry out my own research there, asking me to continue his legacy. Esperanza became the gatekeeper to my work in the village. Because I lived in her home, she introduced me to the issues and concerns the women held and introduced me to the women she thought would best answer the pressing questions I had about their lives in the village.

You will read the stories of some of these "good" and "bad" mothers—labels that the women sometimes applied to themselves, though more frequently such labels were applied by others. Their stories bring into focus the sometimes-conflicted interplay between being indigenous and being a mother. I tell the story of Esperanza, who uncomplainingly manages her household despite constant hip and back pain from a prolapsed uterus.[11] Gloria uses laughter and compassion to overcome the horror of losing a child. Frida and Carmela are two women whose love-hate friendship epitomizes the struggles to find normalcy in their lives as mothers. Alicia and Estela are mother and daughter who somehow manage to care for the five generations of men living under their roof while also bringing up Estela's two young children. Alicia became my *comadre* a few months after we met and was one of my closest friends, while Estela became my most recent *comadre* after I traveled with Rahul, my husband, from the US during my own pregnancy in 2009 so we could serve as godparents to her children.[12]

Juana's kindness and generosity is particularly poignant as she balances the needs of the five of her eight children who are still at home against the vagueness and an itinerant income from an alcoholic husband. Her daughter Camila, who was thirteen when I met her, was my self-appointed assistant until her own unexpected marriage and motherhood at the age of eighteen. Lourdes, the strong, witty, but fragile *partera* (traditional birth attendant), had remarkable knowledge of plants and women's health and had a reputation for being a powerful healer that extended far beyond the borders of the region. She became one of my dearest friends. Ofelia, Lourdes's daughter-in-law, had an unintended pregnancy leading to a fourth child that nearly caused the dissolution of her marriage; she always called me in for a snack as I walked by, and as she plied me with food and drink, we would talk about her eldest daughter's health troubles or her despair over her youngest son's—my godson's—failing first grade. Cristina served me meal after meal as she confided her fears about her youngest daughter's lack of interest in food, and how this might cause stunting and problems later in her life. And Refugio's reputation as a powerful *partera* and healer was marred by accusations of witchcraft, which prompted her to find income-generating projects outside of the village. The voices of these women, along with many others, can be heard in the pages of this book, telling their stories of motherhood, indigenousness, and modernity.

Juana, Lourdes, Cristina, Ofelia, and their families were my neighbors during the time I lived in the small, indigenous Nahua village of Amatlán, in eastern Mexico. Over the course of four field seasons between 2004 and 2007, constituting over fourteen months of ethnographic fieldwork, I lived and learned from the extraordinary women who make their lives in this changing village. In total, I spoke with over ninety people—mothers, husbands, children, physicians, nurses, and teachers.[13] The women's lives I describe here are filled with the joys of motherhood and the tragedies of hardship and loss. These women's lives are not struck by the "everyday violence" described by Nancy Scheper-Hughes (1993) among the women in northeast Brazil—there is plenty of food, the village is relatively auto-nomous in many respects, and their dependence on the largesse of the Mexican state is not terribly dire. These people live normal lives—they are not desperately poor, and they are not starving. Their subsistence, though not luxurious, has not been taken over and destroyed by the regional cash crops, and it provides them with the basic foods—maize, chilies, and squash. Their lives are not those of quiet desperation.

Nonetheless the lives of the women, men, and children of Amatlán are afflicted by the unintended consequences of development, which are coupled with the historical marginalization faced by indigenous groups across Mexico. Health and development policies enacted through programs like Oportunidades, despite their good intentions, may reproduce struc-tural violence—defined as the historically given and economically driven insidious political and economic forces that increase suffering in vulnerable populations. In this situation, people's choices become limited by racism, sexism, political violence, or grinding poverty (Farmer 2006). The presence of structural violence exists in many of the interactions in these women's lives—with medical and economic authorities or with educational institutions. This structural violence is not grinding, nor does it impact their lives in desperate ways. Instead, it is insidious. In some cases, such as in Oportunidades, it filters in through welfare programs intent on "modernizing" and "developing" their lives. And it is the women's motherhood itself that becomes a target for change.

Developing Human Capital: A Look at Oportunidades

It has been very clear in Mexico that the divide between rich and poor, between haves and have-nots, has only increased over the decades of the twentieth and twenty-first centuries. Despite economic upswings, open trade borders, free trade agreements, and remittances sent from abroad, a large proportion of the country's population lives in poverty. Such a situation has been of much concern to the country's leaders and academics, leading to a series of welfare and development programs to aid these populations. Mexican social programs have historically consisted of aid in the form of foodstuffs and staples subsidies, which, according to Skoufias (2005), typically were costly to the government without having much effect at alleviating poverty.

Oportunidades emerged in 1997 as the brainchild of two economists, Santiago Levy and José Gómez de León, who envisioned it as a stopgap, safety-net program to alleviate poverty.[14] Its name literally means "opportunities"—referring to the new opportunities and possibilities that open up for the enrolled families. Specifically, Oportunidades aims to improve human development by focusing on the triad of children's health, nutrition, and education (Levy 2006). It is envisioned to coordinate with other social programs to "promote employment, income, and savings of people in extreme poverty" in order to "propel and strengthen their capabilities and potentials, elevate their standard of living, generate opportunities, and bring about their integration into comprehensive development" (Diario Oficial 2002:10, my translation). This integrated structure reflects a belief that simultaneously addressing all aspects of human capital will bring about greater social returns than their implementation in isolation (Skoufias 2005:2). In 2012 the program celebrated its fifteenth year in existence and continued to be lauded as Mexico's most successful welfare program.

Enrolling more than one-third of the country's population, Oportunidades is the largest social welfare program that Mexico has ever implemented.[15] Combining short- and long-term objectives of extreme poverty alleviation, its mission is to develop "the basic capabilities of people" as well as to improve their "access to economic and social development opportunities" (Secretaría de Desarrollo Social [Ministry of Social Development] [hereafter SEDESOL] 2011). Its goal is that by 2030—more than thirty years after it was first implemented—all poverty will have been eradicated and all Mexicans will have equal social rights and equal access to opportunities.

To achieve the intended improvement and development of the population, a bimonthly conditional cash transfer is made between SEDESOL and the children's mothers.[16] The mothers are given the money directly; there are no intermediaries. All conditional cash transfers (CCTs) are designed so that, as their name suggests, there is a conditional element behind the exchange of money. Money flows from the government to the welfare recipient, while the recipients must follow certain conditions and meet particular criteria in order to receive the money. Operating under the assumption that women are more responsible than men at managing a household, Oportunidades makes women the primary node for the cash transfers. Not unlike other social programs across the globe, the assumption about responsibility lies at the core of Oportunidades, essentializing women as nurturers and caregivers who will abide by the government's conditions for developing human capital.

Oportunidades expects mothers to become involved in their children's lives at three nodes—health, nutrition, and education. The conditionality is strictly enforced, whereby if a mother does not follow through with the conditions, she will be removed from the program and lose the money grants. This program fits in with the women-in-development (WID) approach, which emphasizes the need to integrate women into development policy and practice. It does not seem to take a more nuanced gender-and-development (GAD) view, which aims to challenge the existing gender roles and relations (Reeves and Baden 2000; see also Bedford 2009).

Oportunidades has been used by many countries as a model for addressing poverty and educational limitations (especially for girls) in several countries. Countries as diverse as Brazil (Bolsa Familia) (Adato and Hoddinott 2007), Nicaragua (the now-defunct Social Protection Network), Turkey (Social Risk Mitigation Project) (Adato 2008), Malawi (cash transfers through the Malawi Social Action Fund) (Nigenda and González-Robledo 2005), and the United States (NYC Opportunity, which was cancelled after three years) have implemented conditional cash transfers. Conditional cash transfer programs have also been suggested as a possible way to curb risky behavior, particularly sexual behavior, by encouraging a "healthy behavioral change" to prevent transmission of sexually transmitted infections in sub-Saharan Africa (Medlin and de Walque 2008). The popularity of conditional cash transfers does not necessarily make them the perfect model, and neither does it prove that they are the right way to do things. However, given the influence of this program on poverty-reduction strategies in many parts of the world, it is important to address it in its entirety, particularly the ways the program is experienced by its intended population—the women—and to address their feelings about it, which are often ambivalent.

At the highest national level, it is easy to see such a program harboring well-meaning hopes for the country. But policy is far removed from actual participation in any development scheme. As we encounter actual indigenous mothers, we see the unintended consequences of these programs, in this case, Oportunidades. From a policy perspective, the effects on the women remain invisible, and their fears, concerns, and suffering are ignored. The conditionality of the program places particular emphasis on the responsibility and participation of mothers for the welfare and betterment of their children and, in turn, of the country. If the women fail to follow these conditions, not only might they be removed from the program, but they also are seen as a failure to their children and to themselves. They are marked as disobedient, are removed from the program, and lose their money. Only the obedient ones are good citizens.

"They don't want us to have any more children": *Stratified Mothering*

There has been a long-standing fear in Mexico of the overly reproductive poor, which likely is a remnant of the racialized and gendered vision of European colonial expansion (Sawyer and Agrawal 2000). This view has resulted in the poor sectors of the population becoming irrevocably tied to development and population policies. From the early twentieth century, Mexico's self-conscious will to modernize has pushed the country to restructure its national identity as *mestizo*—mixed ancestry. Indigenous people have historically been purposefully excluded from this identity; all efforts were thus aimed at integrating them into the new Mexico, through various re-education projects. This structure is not unlike other modernizing projects across the globe, such as among rural Chinese women (Chen 2011) or the

Adivasi tribal groups of India (Mahmood 1993), who have been expected to conform to mainstream concepts of modern women and mothers.

Mothers were perceived to be key in Mexico's citizen creation, and so campaigns were launched for hygienic household management and child raising that purposefully targeted indigenous households. The pursuit of modernity in Mexico has become synonymous with adhering to behaviors that promote good citizenship and encourage the country's social and economic growth. In the present day, the nodes of implementation for modernity—and good motherhood—are the many government clinics and hospitals around the country, where women are the recipients of both cash and advice about health and family planning. The cash-for-change approach of the conditional cash transfer programs in which the women are enrolled is little more than a bribe to convince the women to change certain behaviors in exchange for receiving a significant amount of their monthly income. Policies of this sort echo the historical "ideological and geopolitical objectives" (Castro and Singer 2004:xv) of deep fear of the reproduction of certain undesirable groups.

As in many other parts of the global South, the women of Amatlán are caught between wanting to be modern—by giving birth in the hospital and having smaller families—and yet not being fully comfortable with the form of modernity offered to them—with its concomitant lack of medical options, poor treatment at the hands of clinicians, and transformation of social structure in their villages. Scholars of reproductive anthropology have noted the existent tussle between women's concerns and the state's needs. Fordyce (2012) "follows the numbers" to explore how Haitian immigrants' pregnancies have been profiled and categorized as risky by clinicians in Florida. Van Hollen (2003) observes struggles between modernity and local women's birthing traditions in India. Allen (2002) shows the unintended consequences of the implementation of the Safe Motherhood Initiative on local Tanzanian women's reproductive lives. Chen's (2011) work among rural Chinese women brings out notions of modernity and perceived docility. Tapias (2006) shows the effects of neoliberal economic policies on women's embodiment of emotions. Browner's (2000) work among women across Latin America shows that it is the combination of structural factors and cultural processes—particularly the role of male partners—that shape the ways that women's reproduction is situated. Sargent (2005) shows the multiple ambiguities existent between the discourses on the family planning of West African immigrant women in France.

Gender has been central to Mexico's concern with modernity. Using slogans, public relations, and even soap operas, the country has aimed to change the national stereotypical identity of Mexicans from macho men and submissive women to respectful and decisive citizens respectively (Laveaga 2007).[17] There has been great concern with creating the right sort of citizens for the new, modern, less populated Mexico, and the image of the macho, lazy, and irresponsible Mexican man was not deemed to be an advantage. The leaders were searching for "quality" men who did not abandon their homes to become nomadic, itinerant workers far afield. Ironically, none of these government sentiments ever acknowledged the fact that it was government policies that often put men in situations where they had to leave their families to find work and thus become "bad fathers" in the process (Laveaga 2007:24). The government made a similar expenditure of effort to change the Mexican woman from a submissive "baby producer" into a modern woman who "assumes responsibilities and takes decisions over her own life [because] a true woman intervenes, has opinions, decides, participates, contributes . . . and is active" (Laveaga 2007:25). These fundamental changes in the population and the ensuing reproductive decisions reflecting good citizenship became linked to the vision of modern Mexico.

It was especially poor and disenfranchised people who had to be made into good citizens. Women were presented with the "choice" between being pregnant (and poor) or practicing family planning (and being modern). The government never acknowledged the social roots of the attitudes it sought to erase; these roots and causes include poverty, structural violence, historical discrimination, and lack of educational and financial opportunities, among others. Instead, "the slogans implied that these behaviors could be cast off as soon as responsible family planning was embraced" (Laveaga 2007:30). Women across Mexico, particularly the educated middle class, embraced notions of choice within their reproduction and sexuality. Coining the term "voluntary motherhood," they demanded control over their reproductive lives, leading to the legalization of contraception in the 1970s. The discourse of sexual and reproductive health and rights and voluntary motherhood, among other concepts, has permeated programs and policies (at least on paper) since the mid-1990s. Despite these important steps in granting reproductive options for women, modernity for middle- and upper-class women is about choices, whereas for indigenous women it is about submitting to control.

All development policies have unintended consequences; it is inevitable that programs created in sparkling offices far removed from the messy realities of people's lives will have effects that were never foreseen. Some effects—such as a change in people's subsistence and dietary patterns—might not necessarily be detrimental to the program's success. Other effects—such as the diminishing role of traditional healers in people's health—might be detrimental to local populations that unsettle and settle localities (Appadurai 1996). And still others have such significant unintended effects that the program can be deemed a failure, creating new forms of domination and leaving local people further disempowered and disenfranchised. But development—and its associated power and discourse—have been important forces in shaping social reality and produce "permissible modes of being and thinking while disqualifying and even making others impossible" (Escobar 1995:5). Development is a "domain of thought and experience" (Escobar 1995:6) aimed at bringing a state's subjects into modernity. And even if these programs fail, they are likely to be relegated to a shelf in their policy offices of origin—oftentimes simply biding their time until they are dusted off and applied in a different situation down the road.

Over the months I lived in Amatlán, I grew to understand how motherhood, modernity, and indigenousness became entangled in the women's lives. Contradictory definitions of indigenous and low-income women were at play; the women were seen as overly reproductive and disobedient bad mothers by larger institutions, and yet they simultaneously worked themselves to the bone to follow the rules and conditions expected of their motherhood. Throughout the book, I have purposefully differentiated between the terms *obedience* and *compliance* for the women's behaviors. The notion of obedience encapsulates, in a much broader way, how Mexican intellectual and economic elites view the indigenous people. Disobedience goes beyond not complying with clinicians' instructions at medical centers, instead extending into all behaviors associated with a woman's entire reproductive and maternal life. What was apparent in these women's lives was the way that obedience *and* disobedience were simultaneously embodied by the women and projected onto the women's bodies by mainstream Mexico.

The women of this region are generally quite obedient to the rules of the state. Teachers and clinicians would often remark about the women's passivity. This is illustrated by Aurora, the kindergarten teacher of Amatlán, who stated, "I tell the women not to allow themselves to be pushed around." The women are respectful of the (perceived) social hierarchy, and while they might grumble among themselves or privately laugh at some of the indignities that they face in clinics or in their interactions with the larger Mexican state, they often try to follow the rules. Despite physicians and other representatives of the Mexican state frequently seeing the individual women as passive and obedient, this obedience by the women as a group was somehow ignored by the establishment. Indeed, they are more often perceived as *dis*obedient than obedient. This definition of their disobedience is at the root of their personhood and explains many of their interactions with the state. They are seen as disobedient *because* they are indigenous. It is their very nature and ethnicity of indigenousness that marks them as disobedient.

Historically, the indigenous people in Mexico have been seen as a problem, as a pathetic and embarrassing remnant of a glorious pre-Hispanic past. Their ways of life are described alternatingly as quaint or backward. They are a reminder to the rest of Mexico that the country's *mestizo* identity is simply an illusion. These populations' reproduction and their creation of new lives are viewed as problematic if they do not produce new, modern citizens. Hence any form of reproduction the women have is censured because they are producing more *indígenas*. Their wombs are classified as disobedient simply because they are constantly used—as evidenced by the nurse's words. It is this perceived reproductive disobedience that colors the women's interactions with the Mexican state—personified in clinicians and teachers. Most women expressed puzzlement at the anger aimed at them and wondered why "they don't want so many [people] at the clinic."

Because I was a *xinola*,[18] I was permitted to have conversations about adult topics with the women, such as reproduction or motherhood, which would not have been possible if I had been a *muchacha*—an unmarried girl. My status as a married woman made a difference to our interactions.[19] Moreover my own upper-middle-class Mexican background gave me "insider knowledge" about mainstream and elite Mexican attitudes about indigenous Mexico. Carefully navigating my duality, I participated with the women in their lives as mothers. They, in turn, shared their many joys, deep fears, and nagging concerns about their pregnancies, their births, and especially their ideas about motherhood.

Estela, who was twenty years old in 2007 and had two children—two-year-old Yanine and six-month-old Ernestito—was especially voluble about how her mothering choices were viewed by the clinicians. She said to me, as she bathed her squealing and gurgling son in a small plastic tub, "My son was born in Poza Rica. . . . I did not have a *partera* because in the clinic [in Tepatepec] they don't want it like that. . . . They don't like births to take place with a *partera*." After the bath, she sat down on a plastic chair in the breezeway of the house and effortlessly shushed Ernestito's squeals by pulling up her blouse and allowing him to nurse from her breast. She said with some concern, "The [doctor] says that we should stop breastfeeding at six months because [the milk] is spoiled, that it is only water and it is no longer good."[20] Later that day, she reflected about her reproductive life, saying, as she handed Ernestito to her mother, Alicia, who immediately bounced him on her knee, "I am not [practicing] family planning. After he was born they put in the IUD over there in Poza Rica. I did not want it; I wanted to get the implant that goes in the arm, but the woman doctor over there told me I had to leave [the hospital] with something and so they put in the IUD. They did not let me [choose], [the doctor] was very cross. And [my son] also came as a surprise; I wanted to wait until my girl was older and then have another but . . . I only want these; I don't want any more. They are too much trouble. My husband wanted another but I did not. And now I have the IUD, so . . ."

Estela's predicament illustrates the issues that many of the women in my research experienced. There was a surprisingly small number of pregnant women and newborn children in Amatlán during my first two field seasons. The women blamed the low number of recent pregnancies on the staff at the clinic and hospitals, repeatedly saying, "They don't want us to have any more children." They frequently expressed fears about the coercive nature of their interactions with clinicians and wondered whether their own motherhood was somehow a problem. Most of these interactions mirror the larger social structure of Mexico, where certain populations are habitually encouraged and aided to reproduce (Braff 2008), while others—namely indigenous women such as those of my acquaintance—are discouraged in overt and covert ways from reproducing. Kanaaneh (2002:252) observes, "Through the interrelated spheres of national identity, economic strategies, corporeal disciplines, social stratification, and gender relations, modernization has become profoundly entangled with reproduction. Together they create a complex and compelling web of new reproductive discourses and practices through which the modern and the backward are conceived and ranked." This stratified reproduction (Colen 1995) also becomes a form of stratified mothering, where only some women are encouraged to be mothers based on preexisting notions of responsibility and ability. Embedded within the women's reproductive lives—and the interactions that emerge from these lives—are unconscious behaviors and forms of being.

These behaviors are part of the women's *reproductive habitus*—which I refer to here as modes of living their reproductive body, their bodily practices, and their creation of new people through their mothering behaviors. The women in the pages of this book are strong, determined, and humble and—unwittingly and unconsciously—embody a perceived disobedience and do so despite the forces and institutions that expect them to be compliant.

"All this is Amatlán"

Amatlán is in the northern part of the state of Veracruz, in what is commonly known as the Huasteca. The culture area of the Huasteca is a vast geographic, cultural, and economic region that partly covers several states in central-east Mexico—primarily Hidalgo, Veracruz, Tamaulipas, and San Luis Potosí (Lomnitz-Adler 1992). Its limits to the east and west are the Gulf of Mexico and Sierra Madre Oriental respectively. As Ruvalcaba Mercado (2004) points out, the limits of this region have changed significantly over the course of history. This is a land that defies classification. From the rugged, craggy, lush sierras dotted with indigenous hamlets, to the rolling landscape to the east, flourishing with vast, privately owned cattle and citrus farms interspersed with small, communal, indigenous smallholdings, and to the wealthy coastal plain, one of the oil-producing capitals of the country, the area is marked by contrast.

Over the past decade, a considerable amount of research has been carried out in this region, primarily spearheaded by the Centro de Investigaciones y Estudios Superiores en Antropología Social, the Center for Advanced Anthropological Research and Studies (CIESAS), based in Mexico City. This center has particularly promoted ethnographic work by indigenous students and scholars of the Huasteca, contributing to what Narayan (1993:680) calls an enactment of hybridity. Research for this area includes work in archaeology and ethnohistory (Escobar Ohmstede 1998; Pérez Zevallos 1998); agriculture and natural resources (Nava Vite 1996; Ruvalcaba Mercado 1998a); religion, language, and local medicinal practices (Sandstrom 1998; Gómez Martínez 2002; Hernández Bautista et al. 2004; van Hooft 2007); and politics, education, and change (Montoya Briones 1990; Szeljak 2003; Ruvalcaba Mercado 2004).

This area was long seen as peripheral, but in recent years it has received increasing attention from the ecotourism industry. Articles in travel magazines such as *México Desconocido*—"Unknown Mexico"—breathlessly tell its readers, "The Huasteca . . . is a splendorous place because of its sceneries and exuberant vegetation; its rivers and spectacular waterfalls; its caves and deep chasms; [and] of course, because of the magic of its archaeological

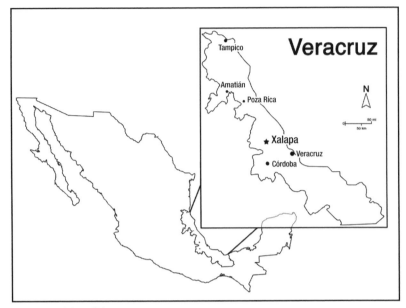

Figure 1.1. Map of Veracruz

sites and the greatness of its ethnic [groups] who, by living their customs and traditions hearken back to a past that is still present in each corner of this fascinating region of Mexico" (2011, my translation). This description illustrates the views held about the Huasteca: it is peripheral, but romantic and exotic. These words are a magnificent example of the ethnographic present being used to promote ethnocultural tourism to witness noble savages living splendidly pristine lives. Not only is such a perception of indigenous people an insult to indigenous and small-scale groups anywhere, but it is also altogether erroneous for the indigenous populations of this region.

The Huasteca in northern Veracruz occupies six thousand square kilometers. This region, of sparse population, also has little infrastructure. The largest city in the Huasteca *veracruzana* is Poza Rica, with just under two hundred thousand inhabitants. The main attractants to the region are the oil business[21] and the archaeological site of El Tajín—a World Heritage Site from the Mesoamerican Classic period best known for its pyramid of niches. Lying to the east of the Sierras, the area receives abundant rainfall because of the warm, moist winds coming over the Gulf of Mexico that release moisture as they cool while rising over the mountains. Most of the rain falls during the wet season (July to November) as violent thunderstorms. In the remainder of the year, very little rain falls, the dryness culminating in May and June—the hottest and driest time of the year. It becomes so hot that it feels as though one's very clothes are burning the skin, and plastic chairs have been known to disgorge the people sitting on them by suddenly becoming flaccid and flexible. The men despair at this time of year, talking about how their maize plants will never grow if the rains do not arrive soon. Of course, when the rains become too strong, especially by the middle of the rainy season, then the worry is that the plants will drown. There is a tight balance needed in the weather for the maize crops to be successful and abundant.

Socially, this area is marked by contrasts. In evidence are some of the highest rates of illiteracy and a lack of services, communications, schools, and jobs in the country, which juxtapose with the "feudal" cattle estates (Ariel de Vidas 2005) of the wealthy landowners who own the majority of the arable land. On the land itself can be seen the stark contrasts between the small-holdings and the ranching estates. These estates produce about 40 percent of the cattle ranching activity of the state, which is in turn the largest cattle producer in the country. Indeed, most of the land surrounding Amatlán that does not belong to indigenous *ejidos* is used for cattle pastures.[22] Cattle equal wealth in this region, and to be a *vaquero*, a cowboy, is a mark of high prestige, especially for the youth intent on upward mobility. No longer are young men content with agricultural labor and the centrality of corn in their production. Instead, men increasingly look to the *vaquero* lifestyle—horses, hat and boots, and *corridos*—from northern Mexico as their ideal modes of life.[23]

High rates of human rights violations, economic exploitation, and oppression by the wealthy landowners are common; this discrimination against the indigenous people dates back to colonial times. In a seemingly contradictory manner, it is also an area where independent indigenous and peasant organizations have acquired (or are striving to acquire) the political strength to peacefully confront the oppression they are facing (Ruvalcaba Mercado 1998b; Szeljak 2003).

Over the years, I have returned to Amatlán countless times, sometimes for long, ethnographic stays and other times for quick, three-day visits to catch up with friends. In this time, I have seen the infrastructure of the region change in marked ways. Most notable in these changes are roads and bridges. When I first arrived in the region, the only way to cross the wide and torrential Vinazco River to reach the municipal head of Ixhuatlán was across a vehicle-wide concrete-and-pylon ford. The base of the ford was not straight across the river; instead it curved up and down, following the gradient of the riverbed. It was often impassable because it was very low along the surface of the river, and as the river water rose during the rainy season, it would cover the ford. Even during low water, vehicles had to drive slowly across each of its jagged humps for fear of toppling over into the swirling water below. During extremely busy times, a long line of cars and trucks would form on either end of the ford, the drivers waiting for oncoming traffic to clear. But by 2007, a shiny new bridge was built, which completely replaced the old ford. The state government instituted several infrastructural projects in the region whereby bridges and paved roads were developed to connect the more remote areas with the market and economic centers. This impetus to push this region into modernity and globalization parallels the state's efforts to bring the mothers into the arms of mainstream Mexico through central government policies.

Amatlán is an extremely small and compact village, with a population of approximately six hundred. The people belong to the Nahua indigenous group; as speakers of Nahuatl, they are the linguistic descendants of the Aztecs. This 468-hectare *ejido* lies in a small valley, surrounded on almost all sides by steep hills. These hills, now mostly denuded of their original forest cover, are used for agriculture or cattle ranching. The rolling landscape is composed of a patchwork of maize fields, cattle pastures, orange groves, and a few stands of extremely scrubby secondary forest.

The village is in the municipality of Ixhuatlán de Madero (see figure 1.1), which has fewer than fifty thousand inhabitants. The Nahuatl etymology of "Ixhuatlán" is "the place of *papatlas*"; *papatlas* are large-leafed plants, very similar to bananas, whose leaves are used to envelop *zacahuiles*—extremely large tamales. The municipality claims its origins at the beginning of the seventeenth century, which is reflected in its colonial-era central church and older buildings. The town obtained its "surname" of "de Madero" after the Mexican revolution, in honor of Francisco I. Madero, one of the revolutionaries who gained support among the townsfolk in the early twentieth century (Nava Vite 2009). Over 70 percent of the municipal population is indigenous, and their primary means of production are small-scale agriculture and cattle ranching (Instituto Nacional para el Federalismo y el Desarrollo Municipal 2011). While most of the population is Catholic, there has been an increase in Pentecostalism over the past two decades (Sandstrom 1991). This religious conversion has brought about significant changes in the lives of the people and in some villages has led to the veritable dissolution of the long-standing pre-Hispanic belief systems.

The people of Amatlán are farmers and have been for many generations. They have historically relied on maize growing, though they are

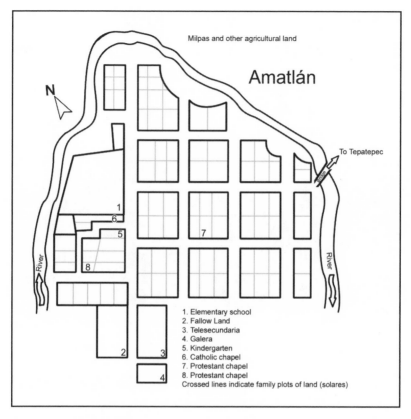

Figure 1.2. Map of the village

increasingly incorporating cattle ranching and orange growing to their subsistence. Maize is their principal crop, around which many other economic and religious activities revolve (Szeljak 2003). Sandstrom (1991) shows the complex way maize plays a central role in people's lives as both food and ritual. As he states, "To call [maize] a staple in the same sense that potatoes are a staple in the North American diet is to underestimate its importance seriously" (132). It sustains people physically and spiritually. Maize provides the underlying structure for the pre-Hispanic pantheon of spirits, saints, and souls that are part of the folk Catholicism of the region. The corn spirit, Chikomexochitl (Seven-Flower) "is both a provider of sustenance and a nourisher of the human soul" (Sandstrom 1991:133), who saved humanity with the gift of food crops, primary of which is maize (Szeljak 2003; Sandstrom and Gómez Martínez 2004). As Nava Vite (2009), a professor at the university in Ixhuatlán de Madero,

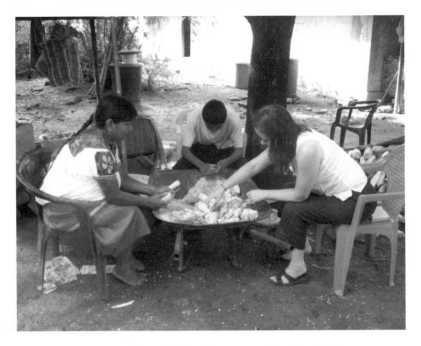

Figure 1.3. Shucking corn from the fields. Photo courtesy of Stephanie Fairhurst

shows in his work on maize consumption and ritual among the indigenous people of Ixhuatlán, maize is perceived to be such a strong nourisher that it allows people to live to ripe old ages of one hundred years or more.

No meal is complete without tortillas; it would be unthinkable to eat anything, even a heavy rice-and-bean soup, without the complement of tortillas. One evening at dinner, Esperanza served the family an enormous pile of *xamitl*—moist, heavy, fresh sweet-corn tamales; she had spent all day making them from scratch. After eating about four *xamitl*, her eldest son asked aggrievedly if that was all the food she had and why had she not made tortillas. It does not matter how full one can get at a meal; it simply is not a proper meal without tortillas. Fortunately, despite the lack of money and the intemperate weather patterns, there is no lack of maize to make tortillas.

My most persistent memories of Amatlán are of the smells—the smell of wood smoke from the cooking fires, the sour odor of the pigsties mixed with the stink of the latrines, the scent of the smoke from burning chicken feathers that acridly catches in the eyes and throat, or the aroma of Esperanza's fresh tortillas cooking on the hot *comal*.[24] The wood-smoke smell sticks with me, yet when I was there I barely noticed it. All the households are fueled by wood fires, where the women cook the meals for the family over the hearth. No hearth is ever cold and can quickly be prodded with some corncobs and wood into a rapid flame, ready to boil some water for coffee or to heat up the *comal* for tortillas. Certain heady aromas quickly take me back to those kitchens in Amatlán, and I can practically taste the strong, sweet coffee and the roasting chilies for the family's *mole* sauce.[25]

Each time I go to the village, I stay at Esperanza and Ildefonso's home, where I am always treated like a member of the family. Both are truly good people. Esperanza is shy and quiet, blessed with an incredible sense of humor. We found the same things funny—a child riding a bicycle three times too big, the dogged insistence of itinerant traders hawking overpriced wares, or her neighbor Hilario's suggestion that I take several swigs of cane alcohol and lemon to get rid of a cold—and would sometimes laugh until tears flowed from our eyes. Her grandson Tito would laugh along with us and would often be the instigator of our laughter. Her husband, Ildefonso, is one of the kindest people of my acquaintance. He exudes kindness and dependability. His gentle smile often plays at the corners of his mouth at Tito's antics; he rarely has a cross word for anyone.

As I am in the same age group as their four children, my role in Esperanza and Ildefonso's home has been that of a daughter. Both of them were exceedingly generous with me, and I would share in their lives as a relative would. On many occasions, especially during the times when I would call Esperanza from the US, she would call me *hija* and ask questions with motherly concern.[26] This care and concern were especially evident when Hurricane Katrina hit New Orleans in 2005. Though Esperanza and Ildefonso knew that I lived in Chicago, they were not entirely sure how far that was from the floods. I received a phone call from my own mother, who said that Esperanza had called her in Mexico City and was very worried about my safety. When I spoke to Esperanza, she asked fearfully if I was all right because she had heard on the news that "the United States is sinking." Her words crystallized the fact that I was a member of the family and that my duties and obligations to her and my other friends and *comadres* in Amatlán were that of a covenant. I was part of the village.[27]

Lourdes the Partera

One of my primary guides during my time in Amatlán was Lourdes. She is a no nonsense woman in her late fifties who gave had given birth to and raised eight children. A slight woman with a ready smile, she carried herself gracefully and always dressed the best she could, in embroidered blouses and long skirts. Samuel is her youngest son, who was sixteen years old in 2004. Lourdes is a healer and traditional birth attendant who works very hard tending her home garden, collecting firewood and carrying water, shucking corn, and walking to nearby villages to attend to patients. She and her husband are extremely poor, and she is always in debt at the village stores, many of which refuse to give her credit until she has paid part of her debt off. She considered the money from Oportunidades to be a godsend, though it never seemed to be enough to help her move out of the cycle of debt she found herself in. She was a jack-of-all-trades, who not only worked professionally as a *partera*, ritual specialist, and *sobadora*, but who also joined any cottage industry available—such as the bakery or a sewing group—to try to make some money and pay off her debts. She was easily the busiest woman in the village.[28]

Lourdes's life has not been easy, having been marked by an extremely deprived childhood. Her mother died when she was very young, and her father "was a *borracho*, a drunk," who contributed nothing to the family welfare. Lourdes was thus obliged to work as a *pijlnana* (a nanny) for a woman who paid her twenty-five pesos a month. She said she used that money to feed her siblings *tochones* (dry, old tortillas) and bean broth. Admitting that she "didn't even have clothes," she said she had only one outfit, which she would daily wash, wring out, and wear again. It was such a desperate situation that led her to marry Rufino at the age of thirteen. She said ruefully, "I was very foolish. I thought that being married would be nice. I could see all the married women and I thought it was nice, but it wasn't [so]. I was a fool."

While Lourdes and Rufino have a companionable marriage, their life has been one of living constantly beyond their means. Their home is made of wattle and daub, with a mud floor, and is little more than ten paces wide. Half the house is used as a living area, with a handmade bed in one corner and with a very intricate altar that shows how actively Lourdes uses it. There are always votive candles burning, fresh bags of dried beans sit on it, and the saints appear well looked after. The other half of her home is a kitchen. Its roof is so low that I can only crouch when I am inside. A pot of aromatic coffee is always warming on the stove, and Lourdes always welcomed me with fresh, warm, moist bread and, despite my entreaties to the contrary, by sending out the nearest child for a bottle of soda. Within her *solar* are also the houses of her sons; they are made of concrete.[29] One even has two floors, though it is still in the construction stage. It belongs to a son who is a policeman in Mexico City.

She is an avid chicken keeper. Many of her patients pay her with chickens, and she loves to collect the ones with the strangest feather patterns—tufted heads, bald necks, or overgrown tail feathers. Her favorite ones have crinkly feathers, which lend the chicken an air of a surprised carnival dancer. She finds the chickens funny and enjoys the odd outcomes from the interbreeding. They and their chicks constantly run underfoot.

Of Lourdes's eight children, only three are daughters. One daughter lives in Amatlán, but on the other side of the village with her parents-in-law. Lourdes's daughter-in-law Ofelia, who is married to her eldest son, lives in the family compound. She is of excellent support to Lourdes, particularly in helping her with cooking. But she also has her own family of four children to feed and look after. Lourdes's sons, especially those working in the city, provide her with some income, but she spends much of her time worrying about lack of money, her chickens, and her children's welfare. She is also borderline diabetic. Her energy and health have declined over the years. She said worriedly one day, "I lack *fuerza* (strength); I lack vitamins. With so much work one gets tired. I need medicine, a treatment." Because of the diabetes and the lack of *fuerza* she is more prone to weakness and thus is frequently ill. Years of hard work and ill health have taken a toll on her body, causing her to suddenly lose a series of teeth. The ill-fitting dentures inserted by the local dentist had the unfortunate effect of reshaping her mouth, visibly aging her.

Despite her troubles, Lourdes is always cheerful and full of jokes. Her wit comes through in her comments about village life and the change in local traditions, referring to the veritable disappearance of the *costumbre* in the face of Pentecostal faiths: "Of course [*costumbre*] won't be done [anymore]! Now it's all just hallelujah."[30] Her knowledge of medicinal plants, especially those to do with reproduction, was encyclopedic, and she knew where to find the best plants for issues ranging from heavy menstruation to displaced uterus, postpartum cleansing, or weakening after birth. Lourdes became one of my dearest friends in Amatlán. We looked after each other's interests. She would share her extensive knowledge about healing, traditional birth attendance, and medicinal plants with me, and she and Ofelia would periodically feed me the best *mole* I have ever tasted, and I was pleased to take on the role of godparent to Samuel when Lourdes and Rufino asked.

Because of my friendships with Lourdes and Esperanza, with Jacqueline and Frida, with Emma and Cristina, and with Alicia and Juana, I learned about the various layers that interplay in these women's lives: their motherhood interplays with their health, their reproductive health interplays with Oportunidades and modernity, and their indigenousness interplays with their citizenship. Though Amatlán is a world onto itself, and it becomes my world whenever I am there, it is all too often just a small, forgotten, and disempowered place buffeted by the forces of economic and health development programs.

CHAPTER I

"Somos Mexicanos":

Giving Birth to the Nation

Mexico Modernizing: Creating a National Identity

THE NINETEENTH CENTURY WAS A TIME OF TREMENDOUS UPHEAVAL for Mexico: it lost almost half its territory to the US in 1848; segregation of the old classes and castes was officially abolished, and vestiges of the colonial period were destroyed; communal landholdings (belonging to both the Church and the indigenous people) were forced to privatize under the 1857 constitution; the War of the Reform between liberals (led by Benito Juárez—an indigenous man from Oaxaca) and conservatives led to a high death toll and deep economic debt; the French invasion of 1863 and the installation of Maximilian of Hapsburg as emperor led to grim outcomes; and Porfirio Díaz—a man of mixed ancestry, a *mestizo*—ruled as a dictator for thirty-five years through a series of reelections (Brading 1988).

Despite the presence of two major political figures with clear indigenous roots—Benito Juárez and Porfirio Díaz—during most of this period, the pre-Hispanic past was romanticized and exoticized, while the indigenous populations were seen as degraded and quaint versions of the past (Warman 1970). The anthropologist Sanz Jara refers to the nineteenth century as the time of "Indian negation" (2009:259). During this period, the national leaders' gaze was firmly set on emulating western Europe and the United States and their ideas of individual interests and an unrestricted market. The indigenous populations were at best ignored and at worst viewed as hindrances to the country's modernization. Their position within the country has historically been precarious. After the colonial period, slavery and segregation were officially abolished, yet the indigenous people still lived a mostly feudal existence under the thumbs of *hacendados* or the lords of the manor. During this period, across the country many policies were set into place to strip the indigenous people of their juridical personalities and to distribute their communal lands to individuals. Additionally, because many indigenous populations were isolated and spoke languages other than Spanish, they could not be defined as Mexican citizens (Brading 1988). It was not until the Mexican Revolution—with its original call to equality and rights for all—that the "Indian"—as a creation of the colonial system—truly disappeared (Warman 1970).

While the area of Ixhuatlán de Madero was peripheral, the feudal state of affairs continued until the early decades of the twentieth century for most of the indigenous communities. Alan Sandstrom's (1991) rich data on the history of Amatlán shows that until the early 1930s, the people of Amatlán lived and worked for an *hacienda* owned by a woman called Felícitas Ramírez de Martínez.[1] There was much violence during this period, especially targeting the indigenous people; Sandstrom notes that this was less to do with the revolution than with land reform. This violence took a toll on the communities. Esperanza recounted what her mother experienced during this period:

> People used to fight and kill each other a lot back then. My mother used to tell me all this when I was little but I paid no attention. I thought I didn't have to know about this. They say that when [my mother] died she was over 110. It seems that they would kill so much back then that when my mother was a little girl they had to sleep in the forest because if not this man would come and he would kill the men and with the women, well, he would do what he wanted with them. So they would go to the forest to sleep. . . . [That man] was called Máximo.

Socorro, an elderly woman in her early eighties who is one of the village's traditional birth attendants, recounted a similar story, whispering,

> In the past this was a small village; it had only a few houses. . . . I saw when Máximo [came to] kill. . . . He brought his henchmen and many horses and he would kill. Men would run away. [People] would put rags in children's mouths so they wouldn't cry. . . . [Back then] there were many hacienda owners. They would screw the men and not pay them. They just [made them] work and they would whip them. They would not feed them. My father [Ignacio] said, "I'm going to solve this even if it kills me; my children will [at least]

be alive." And later they did kill him. . . . And he fixed this village so they wouldn't beat people any more. So that [people] would be happy in their homes and would not run [away]. I was little. I stayed with my mother and [Máximo] showed her his weapon and said, "Where did Ignacio go?" and she said, "I don't know."

Through stories with Esperanza, Socorro, and Don Eladio (the oldest man in Amatlán, who claimed he was a grown man during this violence and who swore that he was over a hundred years old[2]), I gathered that eventually Máximo's violence extended to killing not only the *gente campesina*—indigenous people and farm folk—but also *personas grandes*—important people. This final infraction was the tipping point. He was eventually captured and executed. This marked the end of the violence and the beginning of the land reform for the people in the region.

The Mexican Revolution (1910–1917) annihilated Mexico's image as a solid, monolithic, and progressive country; in its place emerged a violent, multicultural country with deep chasms between its various populations (Warman 1970). The conflict emerged originally as a response from the country's intellectual bourgeoisie (embodied by Francisco I. Madero), who wanted Díaz to share more of his power with them. Díaz's strong refusal sparked Madero to radicalize and, under the slogan *"Sufragio efectivo, no reelección"* (Effective suffrage, no reelection), rose up in 1910. With a call for land reform and indigenous rights, Emiliano Zapata—a peasant farmer from the state of Morelos—joined the fray. He led a hodgepodge of indigenous and peasant guerillas, who clearly confirmed the presence of the marginalized and downtrodden within the war. Several different revolutions were fought during the war's ten years—by Zapata's southern peasants, by Pancho Villa's northern cowboys and railway workers, and by Madero and Venustiano Carranza's urban and middle-class fighters. The latter group eventually gained the upper hand and, drafting a new constitution in 1917, created the core political machine that was to rule Mexico for the rest of the twentieth century.

After the Mexican Revolution, the country was in turmoil economically, politically, and socially; this prompted the postrevolutionary leaders to consolidate the country under one political ideology. They strove to reorganize and modernize the country through innovations in industry, communications and infrastructure, the agrarian sector, and the health and population sectors. Within this process of modernization, the "indigenous question" resurfaced over and over again especially concerning what the population's role and place in the emerging society should be. Various sectors of the ruling society became concerned with the ethnic and national identity of Mexico. They concluded that Mexico's path to progress was through a strong national identity (Sánchez 1999). Needing to create a "deep, horizontal comradeship" (Anderson 1991:7), the nationalism that emerged from the Mexican Revolution was about unity and about homogeneity, that is, *mestizo*—a mixture of all groups within Mexico.[3] *Mestizaje* thus brought the various revolutionary and postrevolutionary factions under the same umbrella. But in order to create a unifying identity, the leaders actively looked to the pre-Hispanic past to reinvent the identity of the Mexican population as the true and rightful descendants of the glorious Aztecs, Maya, Zapotecs, or Olmecs. The aim was to integrate the indigenous people into the new mainstream Mexico while simultaneously reinventing, reassessing, and rescuing the indigenous cultural heritage that was central to *being* Mexican.

In order to achieve this *Mexicanness*, the state had to intervene and set up systems to shape, integrate, and control the population. Controlling people's bodies is an important step in accomplishing this goal. It is achieved through various processes, and as James Scott (1998:82) shows, the architects of a modern nation-state "do not merely describe, observe, and map; they strive to shape a people and landscape that will fit these techniques of observation." Browner and Sargent (2011:11) point out that the census is integral for managing a population, not only as it represents statistics and measurements (see Hacking 1991) about the aggregate population, but also as it draws on specific criteria in order to develop plans to deal with them. Through the enumeration emerging from a census, surveillance of people becomes easier (Foucault 1995), ultimately making them easier to track and manage. And what better way to control the body politic than to keep numerical account of people's individual bodies? Fordyce (2008) and Greenhalgh (2005) refer to this as "following the numbers" in the making of reproductive subjects. Categories of people are created through these statistics and measurement techniques, creating specific identities that are subsequently bound to assumptions, practices, and norms that people are expected to observe and obey. In this view then, the state is not an exploitative entity, nor is it a benign manager; the state acts as *pater familias* and enforces its own legitimacy through both coercion and integration. Barring individual acts of maximization and self-aggrandizement, the state is a stable if clumsy actor that works on the whole despite the activities of its parts (Oka 2008).

States are especially persistent in their creation of a shared identity. Benedict Anderson (1991) demonstrates how the nation-state uses ethnicity as a tool for management. Gellner (1983) connects literacy with ethnic identity and egalitarianism—all these serve to encourage the loyalty of the population. Within Gellner's framework, the declaration *"Somos Mexicanos"* (We are Mexican)—supersedes all other ethnic affiliations within the nation-state. Curiously, the Nahua often refer to themselves as *"Mexicanos"*: their ethnic group and their language are *Mexicano* (see also Hill and Hill 1986). A nation-state places emphasis on the development of a national culture and is uneasy about difference; difference is seen as dissent and, in various cases, as sedition. When the Nahua say *"Somos Mexicanos,"* it takes on a whole different meaning; they are indigenous Mexicans, the descendants of the original inhabitants, and they also appropriate the nomenclature of the Mexican nation as their own. But the indigenous people's being *"Mexicano"* and speaking *"Mexicano"* is quite different from the elite population's being Mexican and speaking Mexican Spanish. While the former might be descended from the original inhabitants of the Americas, it is the latter who determine true national identity and belonging (see also Clifton 1990). Bonfil Batalla (1996), drawing on Anderson's idea of the imagined community, refers to this dynamic as the *México profundo*—deep or real Mexico—being undercut by the *México imaginario*—imaginary, inauthentic Mexico. He saw these as oppositional forces—one a representative of the precolonial populations that have been historically and systematically disenfranchised by the other—which is imaginary because it takes its culture from abroad and refashions it as (fake) Mexican.

Perhaps one of the unique elements of a modern nation-state is that it is constructed around the idea of productive and compliant citizens. Elizabeth Dore (2000), in her work on the transition of Latin America from the nineteenth century to the nationalism and modernization of the twentieth century, problematizes the issue of the state in those historical and cultural contexts. Using a Marxist analysis, she points out that through the use of coercion and by constructing consent, the state can create the "correct" way of organizing society. This method normalizes and naturalizes certain forms of behavior while eschewing or criminalizing others. For this to happen, people's bodies have to be "subjected, used, transformed, and improved" (Foucault 1995:136). This is especially meaningful for issues of reproduction, gender, and motherhood. Browner and Sargent (2011:11) demonstrate that state ideologies are deployed to encourage certain populations (ethnic minorities, immigrants, and so on) to "adopt the lifestyles and values of the dominant society." States achieve this by creating spaces for health, controlling sanitary practices, producing sanitary citizens, and controlling populations. Ultimately, biological citizenship is desired. Through these coercive institutions, the state will decide what is acceptable and what is unacceptable. Such behaviors are frequently shaped by class and ethnicity. As Dore points out, "States establish a quasi-official gender regime by regulating as many aspects of life as they can reach" (2000:8), which includes, among other things, sexual practices, family planning, parenthood and motherhood, marriage, and the family. Chen (2011:39) argues in his work on China that the state sees itself as progressive and responsible in its quest to transform (female) peasants into "docile instruments of its modernity project." It is the agencies of the state, embodied by various institutions, that are "among many disciplining and socializing bodies that interact in intricate, often contradictory ways" within the society (Vaughn 2000:195). These processes have unfolded over the past century and indeed have constructed the ideal narrative for "*Somos Mexicanos*" as well as the detractions and variations of this narrative as problematic for a modern Mexico.

Son Indígenas: *Integrating into the Nation-State*

Under the new ethnic impetus experienced by Mexico, the presence of indigenous groups existing apart from the mainstream society became problematic. The indigenous people were not part of the homogeneous, *mestizo*, and united nation-state. Instead, they were viewed as a stumbling block to development and modernization. The Mexican leaders thus focused on finding a solution to the "indigenous problem" and on how to achieve the ethnic homogeneity that indigenous people's presence impeded. As with the United States, where for the country to address the "Indian problem," the populations had to be studied, to learn, as Hinsley put it, "how to make [them] other than what [they were]" (Purcell 1998:262), Mexico sought to find ways to integrate and eradicate indigeneity for the racial welfare of the nation. The primary goal became how to integrate the indigenous populations into the national ethos and make them part of the modernizing state. The *indigenous* problem was thus viewed as a *national* problem. This led to the development of *indigenismo*—a politically embedded process for contextualizing and academically "knowing" the indigenous populations. The political underpinnings of *indigenismo* shaped the ongoing marriage of anthropology and development to bring "*los pobres inditos*" (the poor little Indians) into the "*Mexicano*" mainstream.

Indigenismo is inherently contradictory. It emerges from efforts to homogenize the population through cultural *mestizaje;* yet for the establishment to achieve this, the indigenous people had to be studied and understood. The result of this process was to "de-Indianize" the indigenous people while simultaneously exalting the pre-Hispanic indigenous past (Sanz Jara 2009:260). Arturo Warman (1970), one of Mexico's preeminent anthropologists, in a somewhat vitriolic article he wrote almost forty years ago, provides a concise chronology of the disappearance and reinvention of the indigenous people. He states that, while there was consensus that the indigenous populations posed a problem to development, there was little agreement about how the problem could be solved. Many politicians and academics considered the problem racial; the moderates advocated for biological mixture, while the extremists favored extermination and replacement of the indigenous people with European immigrants. Others thought it was an educational problem, which could be solved through a decent western, secular, and free education. Still others thought the problem was poverty, whose solution was charity. As time passed, many scholars and policy makers began to think of the "indigenous problem" as an economic problem: the Indian would remain a problem as long as he did not have a profitable trade, and only through that occupation would he gain access to civilization. The main issue was that "the Indian question[ed] the very existence of the nation" and did not allow it to be a unified entity (Sanz Jara 2009:262).

Sanz Jara (2009) identifies at least two distinct phases of *indigenismo* and a possible third. The first phase runs from 1920 to 1940 and establishes the academic and theoretical base for the ideology; the second is from 1940 to 1960, during which *indigenismo* is put into practice and institutions are created to achieve the transition from what I refer to as "*son indígenas*" to "*somos Mexicanos*"—"they are indigenous" to "we are Mexicans." The decades after 1960 are not quite a phase as much as a transitory muddle. Sanz Jara points out that during this period, there was a lack of theoretical development of the "indigenous"; instead proponents spent their time fending off the attacks of detractors while the institutions atrophied. By the 1960s, with the Cultural Revolution, student movements, and the Tlatelolco student massacre in 1968, many fissures began to emerge within this ideology. Critics of these *indigenismo* policies abounded, including Rodolfo Stavenhagen and Guillermo Bonfil Batalla, both anthropologists and strong advocates for indigenous rights. Even so, integrationist *indigenismo* remained in effect in Mexican policies until the 1980s in one form or another, as a Band-Aid set of remedies, even as the marginalization of the indigenous communities continued unchecked. This ongoing indifference to the realities of marginalization—even as policies continued to pay lip service to national unity and integration—resulted in the final and official disintegration of *indigenismo*.

The final blow to official *indigenismo* occurred at the hands of the Zapatistas, who rose up against the North American Free Trade Agreement on January 1, 1994. With their strong indigenous core and pleas for social justice, the Zapatistas pushed the image of the indigenous people front and center for the Mexican population. The indigenous people were no longer going to be ignored. I was a high school student in Mexico City during this uprising. While the indigenous people and the Zapatistas were suddenly visible in the media, the response to their plight from middle- and upper-class society—who rule the country and implement policies—was not favorable. The sudden visibility of the indigenous population brought to the surface all the hidden opinions people had had of "*los indios*," which until that point had politely been left unsaid, with people speaking only patronizingly about "*los pobres inditos*." The Zapatistas caused the contained racism to explode, and people no longer held back from making racial ad hominem attacks on the indigenous people and the "problems" they brought the nation[4]—echoing early-twentieth-century rhetoric about the country's pathway to modernity and development, and the role indigenous people were to play.

Not long after I finished my fieldwork, I was at a dinner party in Mexico City where most of the attendees belonged to the country's economic and intellectual elite. When I described my research and findings, one of the men dismissively questioned the use of indigenous medical knowledge; despite my efforts to contextualize the historical and social role played by local forms of knowledge, his refrain was that these people's ideas were backward and were in need of modernizing. Such comments show a (perhaps) willful blindness to the fissures and cracks present in modernizing efforts and how easily some blame the indigenous people for their own subjugation.

The Curious Role Played by Anthropology in Indigenismo *and Mexico's Development*

The creation of the Mexican national identity was not solely a political endeavor. Scholars and academics played an important role in developing "Mexicanness," and in how the classification of the population was to function. Their main focus was to develop the ideology and practice of *indigenismo* and decide how to incorporate indigenous people into mainstream culture. Among the main players who helped to usher in this new facet of Mexican life were the anthropologists Manuel Gamio, Alfonso Caso, and Gonzalo Aguirre Beltrán; the philosopher and lawyer José Vasconcelos; and the philosopher and labor leader Vicente Lombardo. Their aim was to homogenize the country's cultural and ethnic makeup to match the dominant society and in turn modernize the country. Liberal and progressive, most of these scholars advocated for the rights of indigenous people. They were the only ones who were concerned about the indigenous populations at all, without dismissing them as the rest of the country's elite classes did. Their approach was to Mexicanize and normalize the indigenous people and "mobilize their disparate energies toward a common goal" (Gamio 2010:28) by understanding their traditional culture better. In the process, the indigenous person was reinvented as something exotic, as "the other." Manuel Gamio illustrates their concerns:

> Can 8 or 10 million individuals of indigenous race, language, and culture hold the same ideals and aspirations, have the same goals, revere the same *patria* [homeland], and treasure the same nationalistic sentiments as 4 to 6 million persons of European origin who inhabit the same territory but speak a different language, belong to another race, and think in accordance with the teachings of a different culture or civilization? We think not. [Gamio 2010:27]

The classification of the indigenous people as not true Mexicans was often based on their lifestyle; they were seen as living in isolation and, as Caso would put it, "stifled by archaic social conditions," people whose culture was "useless and damaging in the modern world" (Sanz Jara 2009:261, my translation).

Like colonial anthropology in the United States or Europe, anthropology in Mexico is a curious animal. From its beginnings in the early twentieth century, anthropologists have had ties to the state and its needs. Gamio saw anthropology as a central part of good government because "through anthropology one knows the population which is to be governed and for whom the government exists" (González 2004:142). Because the government's interests were unification and nationalism, these also became the goals of the anthropological discipline. Roberto Gonzalez (2004) notes that in Mexico, the theory and the practice of anthropology have never been separate entities of the discipline and have both in fact been tightly woven into the fabric of Mexican politics. Warman (1970:34) states, somewhat caustically, that Mexican anthropology "has always served the colonizer" rather than the marginalized. Over time, and through this close connection between academia and governance, the science of anthropology gave way to the skills in implementing the projects and interests of the state. Anthropologists including Manuel Gamio[5] stepped into this role with ease—as they had the tools and methods to understand cultures in great depth. Gamio's definition of indigenous—those people who maintained a high proportion of pre-Hispanic cultural traits in their current lives (León-Portilla 1962)—was central to the government's efforts at integration. Additionally, the Mexican state had acknowledged the important role that anthropology could play in developing the country, and officials encouraged anthropologists to take important roles in government. For much of the early to mid-twentieth century, anthropologists were firmly entrenched in the bureaucratic system. Anthropologists were viewed as the ideal educators who could scientifically "Spanish-ize, alphabetize, and technologize the indigenous" (Warman 1970:30–31, my translation). In doing so, anthropologists had become, perhaps unwittingly, the handmaidens of *indigenismo*.[6]

In the next few paragraphs, I introduce some of the key issues that academics grappled with in their efforts to shape the emerging modern Mexican ideology. Most of the scholars involved in this process were part of the Mexican intellectual elite and, as such, saw themselves as the architects of a new and modern Mexico. As part of the country's bourgeoisie, many of them had a close connection to the builders of the modern Mexican nation and thus held a particular vision of where the country should go.

One of the most influential thinkers during this time was the philosopher José Vasconcelos. Vasconcelos is best known for creating the oft polemicized, and, some would argue, racist, concept of *raza cósmica*—the cosmic race. He saw Latin America as the new cradle for global modernity because its population was a mixture of all four main "races" (European, African, Asian, and Native American). This mixture would create the fifth race, the cosmic race, which, taking the best elements from each group, would become the vanguard of the modern world (Vasconcelos 1925). His ideas created the impetus for *mestizaje* policies to be implemented across Mexico. Out of these ideas emerged the drive to unify the country through integration (Marentes 2000). *Mestizaje* was conceived of as an exchange between cultures: the indigenous population would incorporate by accepting "positive" western values—economy, language, science and technology, political organization, and "Manifest Progress" (Warman 1970:27). In turn, the nation would absorb the "positive" indigenous values—art, sensitivity, and, of course, history. From this meeting of cultures, values, and races, the "cosmic race" would emerge, leading to a strong and balanced nation.

Language became one of the primary markers of Mexicanness. Vasconcelos, as minister of public education from the 1920s onward, helped to establish free monolingual (that is, Spanish) schooling, whose goals were linguistic and cultural unity and the strengthening of nationalism. He created rural schools to promote community development as well as a national conscience and civilization (Sánchez 1999). Such schools were envisioned as nodes for imparting positive western values and uprooting negative values arising from tradition (Warman 1970). Not only did a unified language have a practical purpose, but as Gamio writes, it would lead to a beautiful literature that would revive the "national soul" (2010:113) and contribute to the continued development of a Mexican homeland.

Perhaps because the indigenous populations lived far from cities, concern began to be shown for their communities as such and how they should be defined. Should there be self-determination? Or should the communities be integrated completely, and irrevocably, into Mexican political and social divisions? Vicente Lombardo in particular struggled with this question. Originally his thinking—influenced by Stalinist and Soviet ideas after a visit to the USSR—emphasized the current marginalized state of the indigenous populations, which he termed "oppressed nationalities." Highlighting how past and present policies had shaped their position in society, he took a beginning step toward acknowledging the role of the conquest of the Americas in stripping the indigenous inhabitants of their rights and autonomy. But bowing to strong pressure from Mexican leaders, he rejected this nascent idea of indigenous nations and began to espouse Mexican integrationism where the nation was to be formed solely by true Mexicans and no other (Sánchez 1999). Lombardo began using the term "indigenous communities," which were populations marked by a common territory and language, a similar economy and worldview, and a similar attitude toward the rest of the country. Gonzalo Aguirre Beltrán, an *indigenista* anthropologist and a disciple of Melville Herskovitz (Campos-Navarro 2010), was heavily influenced by Lombardo's ideas, as is evident in his effort to understand the marginalization of the indigenous living in "regions of refuge."[7]

Indigenismo for Aguirre Beltrán was a means for indigenous people to liberate themselves from the asymmetrical relationship their locations had with the elite and urban populations. For this reason, when the Tarahumara of northern Mexico petitioned for legal recognition, Aguirre Beltrán supported the government's denial, arguing that such recognition of a "tribal government" would be a step backward in the political evolution of a developing country (Sánchez 1999:49). Lombardo, however, espoused the opposite idea, which was that the traditional government in indigenous communities had to be respected, and he advocated for the creation of homogenous indigenous municipalities. Aguirre Beltrán disagreed, stating that reservations would isolate the indigenous groups and would not allow their integration.[8] Lombardo maintained that through these steps, these populations would no longer be (over)ruled by *mestizo* and white populations that had no vested interest in indigenous needs (Sánchez 1999). Indeed, many years later this same idea was proposed by President Ernesto Zedillo's government in 1996 as a response to the demands of the Zapatistas for autonomy and self-determination.[9]

Many of the issues with nationalism in Mexico at this time were about modernity, and the place of the indigenous population in the emerging nation. Most of these scholars and crafters of the nation-state advocated heavily for the equality of the indigenous population within modern Mexico. Indigenous equality, Aguirre argued, could be achieved only by making modernity (in all its forms) accessible to the indigenous people, especially those living in regions of refuge (Sánchez 1999). His efforts were aimed at homogenizing cultural traits to minimize economic exploitation of the indigenous populations (Gonzalez 2004). Gamio's approach centered on redressing the historically produced economic imbalance and "substitut[ing] the deficient cultural characteristics of these masses for those of a modern civilization using, naturally, those that exhibit positive values" (Sánchez 1999:30, my translation). The conversion of indigenous people into modernity would be achieved through dissolving their political and economic systems as well as through the creation of lines of communication (roads, radio, and eventually television) to link the peripheral villages with the core towns and cities. Decades later, this same sentiment was echoed by former president Vicente Fox's government, which encouraged the building of roads and bridges in remote areas, such as where Amatlán is, "to ensure that the fruits of globalization reach all corners of Mexico."[10]

With the creation of the Instituto Nacional Indigenista (National Indigenist Institute—INI) in 1948, the state-sponsored acculturation was institutionalized and strengthened. It had several functions revolving around identifying "problems related to the indigenous" groups and "studying the improvement measures required" by these groups (Comisión Nacional [CDI] 2008a:1, my translation). This top-down approach illustrated the effort to place the indigenous population on the path to progress through their integration. The control over the indigenous population was supposed to exist only until "the community has accepted the indispensable cultural changes." Only when the indigenous population had been placed onto the path of integration would their subjection (hypothetically) end (Sánchez 1999).[11]

With the Zapatista uprising of 1994, however, the indigenous people were thrust into public view, making them political subjects that needed to be taken into account (Sanz Jara 2009). Thus, pressure from the burgeoning indigenous emancipatory pride emerging from the uprising precipitated the dissolution of the INI by 2003. Its name, missions, and functions were restructured into the Comisión Nacional para el Desarrollo de los Pueblos Indígenas (National Commission for the Development of Indigenous Peoples, CDI). The commission's aims seem to be somewhat different from integrationist *indigenismo*. Instead, the commission aims to "orient, coordinate, promote, support, encourage, [and] monitor and assess programs, projects, strategies, and public actions for the integral and sustainable development" of indigenous populations according to the Mexican constitution (CDI 2008b:1, my translation). Through the Zapatista uprising and the new CDI emerged the opportunity for indigenous people to regain self-determination and autonomy, which would allow them to once again be considered indigenous *peoples*. The anthropologist Margarita Nolasco states that the Zapatista uprising forced the Mexican government to see the indigenous population as social subjects who were important both for national security as well as for the sustained and general development of the country (Nolasco 2003).

While we can retrospectively criticize Gamio's ideas, and those of his contemporaries, for being racist, eugenic, or culturally genocidal, they were bound by their time, as we are. Indeed, their ideas were often extremely progressive and drew from what was considered scientific truth in much of Europe and the US at that time. Their departure from the nineteenth-century practice of ignoring the cultural minorities to one of helping them to develop and become part of the nation were ahead of their time. What can be considered problematic, from our twenty-first-century point of view, is the transformation of these beliefs and practices—sometimes without modification—into policies over the subsequent decades, whereby even during the present day, the indigenous population continue to be considered a hindrance to modernity and development. Despite the presence of the National Commission for the Development of Indigenous Peoples, much of the country's ideology revolves around *mestizaje*—which inevitably creates a binary opposition of *mestizo*-modernity and indigenous-backwardness. The term "*raciclasismo*," a beautiful combination of *racism* and *classism* coined by a Mexican blogger in late 2011, encapsulates the Mexican elite classes' concerns and attitudes toward poor, indigenous, rural, and, especially, dark-skinned people.[12]

Much has changed over the past few decades in Mexican anthropology. Most anthropologists nowadays are strongly critical of the government and have made notable strides to strengthen the discipline and its academic contributions (see for instance Arizpe 1993; Bartolomé and Barabas 1999; Ariel de Vidas 2005; Hernández Castillo 2001; Medina 1996; Ruvalcaba Mercado 1998b; Smith-Oka 2009). Very few of these anthropologists would consider themselves to be colluding with the state and its interests. As Rodolfo Stavenhagen (1997), an anthropologist-sociologist who is primarily known for his research in agrarian politics and indigenous rights, stated the *indigenista* policies, while well intentioned, were in reality extremely ethnocidal and, considering their objectives of integration, surprisingly inefficient. Yet as Guillermo Bonfil Batalla (1996) stated, indigenous people have consciously maintained their indigenous identity and resisted the government's efforts to integrate and culturally eradicate them. He points out that they have not resisted change as immovable objects, but that they have instead adopted the changes they deem necessary to remain indigenous yet continue to be part of the modern nation. The indigenous populations are not to be discounted but rather have emerged as political and active subjects. Anthropologists nowadays have shifted their focus on the processes of structural violence that keeps indigenous people in greater economic disadvantage.

The legacy of *indigenismo* continues to be present in many Mexican policies aimed at the rural and indigenous populations of the country. The state has certainly not buried *indigenismo;* it has simply refashioned it and embedded it into new projects over the years—from education to health care, population control, and family planning. The myth of the unified, *mestizo* country remains to this day, with the Mexican government continuing to be concerned with development and with the role the rural and indigenous populations play within a developed Mexico. The cash transfer program Oportunidades is an excellent example of the confluence of these various concerns with population and development in current Mexico.

Development in Present-Day Mexico

In the latter half of the twentieth century, Mexico's concern with development was closely connected to population growth and dynamics. Beginning in the 1960s, and following Western policies stating that overpopulation was the primary cause of poverty and instability in the Third World and that contraception was important for development, the Mexican government created several policies to encourage family planning. These policies have been retooled and refashioned over the years, but they continue to retain the ideological concern with the connection between large populations and poverty. Indeed, Arachu Castro (2004) indicates in her work on a public hospital in Mexico City that the integration of reproductive health services, while aimed at improving women's health, frequently reproduced and exacerbated existing inequalities. Despite Mexico's concern with population control, policies have practically ignored male involvement, making men at best an afterthought (Gutmann 2011), as though they are somewhat involved in reproduction but have little to do with family planning. Reproduction is a highly politicized aspect of people's lives, and addressing it opens the door to an increase in social surveillance and regulation of reproductive practices and an increased control of people's body politic, within the idea of a modern state.

Oportunidades is one such program that places surveillance over the enrolled women's body politic. It was established a few years before the Millennium Development Goals (MDG) of the United Nations, yet it has similar goals. These goals have developed and matured from the International Conference on Population and Development (ICPD) held in Cairo in 1994. The MDGs, officially established in 2000, are aimed at improving social and economic conditions in the world's poorest countries; they target a tripartite set of factors—human capital, infrastructure, and economic and social rights. There are eight goals: (1) to eradicate extreme poverty and hunger, (2) to achieve universal primary education, (3) to promote gender equality and empower women, (4) to reduce child mortality rate, (5) to improve maternal health, (6) to combat major diseases, (7) to ensure environmental sustainability, and (8) to develop a global partnership for development.

The first five goals match up very closely with the goals of Oportunidades. The MDG3 and MDG5 are particularly significant to the role that women and mothers have within development and to how they are targets of certain forms of development approaches. The ICPD and the MDG aim to reduce poverty by targeting various aspects of people's lives; the creators acknowledge that people's poverty and related factors are shaped by various constraining circumstances, which need to be addressed in a unified manner.

It is important to point out that the MDGs are not without critics. Saith (2006:1167) states that they "envelop you in a cloud of soft words and good intentions and moral comfort; they are gentle, there is nothing conflictual in them; they are kind, they offer only good things to the deprived." Additionally, "they give well-meaning persons in the north-west a sense of solidarity and purpose [and] they provide a mechanical template of targets and monitoring indicators aptly suited to the limits of the bureaucratic mind." Cornwall and Brock (2005) argue that these are "time-bound, numerical targets" that "imply, rather than direct, necessary policy change." They add that they are "the ultimate in compromise, the lowest common denominators of legitimate change, the price of international coherence and co-operation" (1050). Most critics agree that the MDGs' primary failing is their inability to address the issues of structural inequality.[13]

Other development approaches—for instance microfinance and microcredit or conditional cash transfers (such as Oportunidades)—differ from the larger projects mentioned above. These programs are purely economic in their thinking: if we give people loans, they will make things, and they will have more money, and so they will move out of poverty; or, if we give people conditional money to go to school and receive health and nutritional care at clinics, their education and health will increase. Lamia Karim (2008:14) refers to the lauded microcredit system in Bangladesh as a way to link the "out-of-the-home entrepreneur" with the ideology of neoliberalism where to call one's self poor is pejorative. The primary concerns of such programs are thus with the neoliberal discourse of self-help, responsibility, individual capacity building, and the development of human capital.

Neoliberalism has been a major focus of Mexico's drive to modernize. In the early 1980s, while in the throes of an economic crisis, Mexico reorganized itself through structural adjustment programs aimed at neoliberalizing the economy. Central to the idea of structural adjustment is conditionality[14]—encouraging economic growth by linking financial assistance to following a set of conditions recommended by multilateral bodies such as the IMF or World Bank. In response to this change, Mexico cut social services, particularly to health, education, and nutrition. Women were disproportionately affected by these policies: they worked in low-wage and lower skill sectors and received lower wages than men. Rural regions were impacted the most during this time. The number of people in extreme poverty rose, and the income gap became wider (Alarcón-González and McKinley 1999). The World Bank, possibly influenced by Amartya Sen's capabilities approach,[15] shifted their strategy in the mid-1990s to the Human Development Index, which focused on nutritional status, educational attainment, and health status (Pender 2001). Mexico took this new approach and, reimagining it for the issues plaguing the country, reinjected conditionality and recreated it to be the social structural adjustment program known as Oportunidades.

In a Land of Opportunity

"She comes [to these meetings] because now the [government] gives her [Oportunidades] money. She comes to work. In the past, when they didn't give her, she didn't come." Though Esperanza was referring to her relative who had recently begun to receive money from Oportunidades, her words could have described any of the women in the village. All the enrolled women participated in the expected activities of Oportunidades in exchange for the conditional cash transfers they received bimonthly.

For the women in the municipality of Ixhuatlán, news about the imminent arrival of the money would be imparted by the *promotora* for each village.[16] The money would come to a cluster of villages, with one of the villages chosen as the receiving node—this node changed every cycle, so women would sometimes receive money in their own village, and in other months they would have to go to a neighboring one instead. In order to receive the money, the women would have to show their voting card to prove their identity. The clerks from Oportunidades would drive into the village surrounded by a heavily armed police escort, reminiscent of the money-bag coaches of the Old American West. The armed escort was greatly needed, as the amount disbursed at one time might be close to US$25,000, a king's fortune in this region, which can attract an armed heist. As Esperanza told me a couple of days before one of the occasions the money was to be handed out in the village,

> They are going to bring about twenty policemen because the last time they gave out the [Oportunidades money] some women went to Ixhuatlán to get the money and when they were coming [back] they were stopped and robbed and they lost that money. And the [Oportunidades] people have also been robbed. Because everyone knows beforehand when [the money] will be given out. So now they told us not to tell anyone so that it is not robbed. So now they will come with many policemen.

This turned out to be a wise decision, as a few months later, in July 2004, several masked men tried to rob one of the Oportunidades convoys. The robbers fled into Amatlán on their way to the highway. The police chased them down and captured them, but not before they had a shoot-out

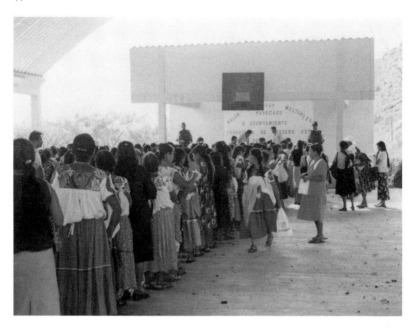

Figure 1.4. Women lining up to receive money from Oportunidades

in the streets of the village. Most people, on hearing the gunfire, ducked into their homes, only occasionally peering out and nervously calling to neighbors to see if they knew if the danger was over. We heard later that Ofelia's eldest daughter, Alana, fainted in shock after witnessing much of the violence while she was at the secondary school.

To avoid such violent situations, in the past few years the government has aimed to create new ways of disbursing the money. Some communities now receive their money via a bank transfer, which opens up the possibility of saving their money (SEDESOL 2011). But with the closest bank being in Alamo, just over an hour away by fast car, two hours by slow bus, this system poses a problem for the people of Ixhuatlán de Madero.

The stipends for children are determined by the sex and year in school of the child: girls receive more than boys (after secondary school), and older students receive more than younger ones. For 2003, the amount for a child in third grade (when the cash transfers begin) was 105 pesos for both girls and boys (which increased to 150 pesos by 2011). For the first year of secondary school (seventh grade) the amounts were 300 pesos for boys and 315 pesos for girls (increasing to 440 pesos and 465 pesos by 2011 respectively). By the last year of school (twelfth grade), the amount for girls was more than doubled (to 655 pesos), and it was just under double (575 pesos) for boys (SEDESOL 2003; SEDESOL 2012a)[17]. The almost 100 peso difference between girls and boys is expected to encourage increased education for girls. For many families in Amatlán, this money amounted to between one-third and one-half of the family's income. While the money was a godsend for Gloria, it never seemed to be enough. She complained, "I get money from Oportunidades, but only a little bit; my boy only receives 240 pesos.[18] With that he buys clothes, school supplies, his shirt, shoes. But everything is already very expensive. Clothes are expensive." She added that she considered her children's money to belong to them, but that she sometimes had to borrow from them to pay expenses. "Everything I have is *fiado*, on credit," she said, and as soon as she receives Oportunidades money she pays off her tabs across the village. She is loath to borrow and beg, though. Comparing herself favorably to Frida, she said she never had to borrow and beg for everything as she did, as she had too much pride.

By 2011 families nationwide received an additional monthly amount of 285 pesos for nutritional support; they also received nutritional supplements (as needed) (SEDESOL 2012a). Students graduating from high school received a one-time lump sum that could be used for additional studies, beginning a small business, building a home (or improving an existing one), and "guarantee[ing] their health and that of their families" (SEDESOL 2003:33). When I spoke with one of the directors of SEDESOL in Mexico City in 2004, this program addition had only just been implemented. It was seen as a way to celebrate and recognize a student's hard work in school. At that time the amount was approximately 900 pesos per graduate, though by 2011 it had increased to 4,192 pesos (SEDESOL 2012a)[19].

Oportunidades is a straightforward program with simple and clearcut goals. Because of Mexico's long history of clientelism and paternalism between the wealthy classes and the poor, urban, and rural populations, and between *mestizo* and indigenous populations, this program is seen as a means to counter what Scheper-Hughes refers to as "hierarchy and dualism" (1993:80). And yet, as Jaime Pensado, a historian of the politics of Mexican student movements, stated, clientelism has also been a form of political participation. It comes from below as well as from above, allowing those in power to meet the needs of the political base (Jaime Pensado, personal communication, April 13, 2012).

An important feature of Oportunidades is that, in contrast to previous government programs, this is touted as an apolitical program not tied to

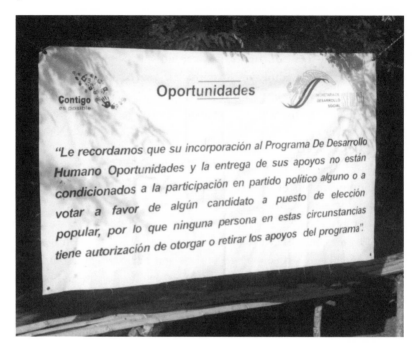

Figure 1.5. Banner for Oportunidades: "We remind you that your enrollment in the Oportunidades Human Development Program, and the receipt of your support, are not conditional upon your participation in any political party or voting for a particular candidate to an elected position. For this reason no person in these contexts is authorized to grant or remove program support."

any particular party, meaning it should not be used to obtain citizens' votes and allegiance (see figure 1.5 above). Though, as Díaz-Cayeros et al. (2006) argue, this ideal vision is far from the local reality, as social assistance programs were used heavily in Mexico during the 2006 presidential elections to buy votes.[20] Fabiola was always heavily involved in politics; one day in 2004, she was trying to gain support to bring a candidate for municipal president to come to speak to the women. She put it quite succinctly when she said, "I always vote for the PRI, because it has supported us. . . . I don't have Procampo but I do have [Oportunidades], and that comes from the PRI. . . . The PRI has always supported us; so win or lose I always vote for it."[21] Over my years in Amatlán, I heard many women echo these words, associating political boons with the PRI, rather than with any other political party. These sentiments show that, though in essence Oportunidades is meant to be apolitical, because of the history of political patronage and clientelism in Mexico, most people continue to associate government assistance with a political party—and will favor one party over another based on these assumptions.

A Look at Other Conditional Cash Transfers

At least on paper, Oportunidades is aimed at helping families to improve the education, health, and nutrition of their children. It uses cash transfers to households, linked to regular school attendance and health clinic visits to accomplish this. The vision is that families living in poverty are aware of the benefits of education, health care, and nutrition but cannot afford the monetary or opportunity costs of such investments in their children.

Situating Oportunidades within international trends, one can see how some countries are using cash transfer programs in an intensive way—oftentimes to achieve Millennium Development Goals. For example, Brazil's Bolsa Familia purposefully aligned itself with the MDGs, particularly those to do with education (MDG2), maternal health (MDG5), and child health and nutrition (MDG1 and MDG4), by strategically targeting those issues in their conditional incentives (Lindert 2006). Honduras saw a significant increase in prenatal care of mothers in poor households when conditional cash was used (Borghi et al. 2006). Among Malawian girls receiving conditional cash transfers to stay in school, researchers saw additional effects regarding a decrease in their rates of sexual activity and early marriage (Baird et al. 2009). In the meantime, other countries, such as the US, the UK, and Canada, are scaling back on social welfare programs altogether. Indeed, this is one of Saith's (2006) main critiques against the MDGs, wherein development is ghettoized to the Third World, ignoring the equally pressing needs of poor people in wealthy countries.

The logic behind conditional cash transfer programs is that poverty can be combated and social inclusion can be fostered by providing poor families with monetary incentives to change certain (seemingly) risky behaviors. The driving ideology is that poor families do not invest enough in basic necessities, a behavior that keeps them in perpetual poverty. The state thus invests in the human capital of the population by paying poor people to engage in modernizing behaviors. Additionally, local consumption receives a boost without undercutting local producers (as food programs often do) (see Molyneux 2007).[22] Karim (2008:12) refers to the emphasis on rural populations for development as a process of "reterritorializing" them for market-driven democratization.[23]

The application of a CCT approach to sexuality is particularly interesting, yet troubling. The main focus of such an application has been on increasing the education and school attendance of girls, with the underlying belief that both schooling and an increase in income lead to a reduced risky form of sexuality; this change is believed to result in reduced levels of HIV and other STI transmission (see Jeffery and Basu 1996 for an opposing view on the correlation between girls' education and empowerment). These projects are seen as "win-win programs" (Baird et al. 2009) as they both increase schooling for girls and reduce their risk of contracting HIV. Many other projects exist that use conditionality to modify women's sexual and reproductive behaviors. Mauldon (2003:361) discusses the ethics of Project Prevention in the United States, which gave financial incentives to drug-addicted women to receive contraception or sterilization. She states that this program "is an attempt at the margins to remedy a larger failing of society and of public policy." Thornton (2003) discusses an experiment she designed in Malawi to provide incentives for people to get tested for HIV—she argues that these incentives not only increased testing but also the purchase of condoms. In Medlin and de Walque's opinion, (2008:12) CCTs could be used to ensure that at risk populations remain free of STIs "that are prevalent within the population, have been incontrovertibly linked to risky sexual activity, and can be easily treated and cured." They suggest a particular focus on prevalent infections such as chlamydia, gonorrhea, or trichomoniasis.

The problem with such cash transfer projects is that they focus on populations that are marginalized and "at risk" but they deal with symptoms of the larger structure, rather than the structures that place them at risk to begin with. They also take the Oportunidades conditionality to a questionably coercive point and border on targeted reproductive control and eugenics. In these cases, the state has created a repressive means to maintain the body politic in place.

The question remains, however, how does a conditional cash transfer program that invests in social welfare make sense in countries such as Mexico or Brazil that are intent on neoliberalism and free trade? The answer might lie in the fact that the underlying structure of Oportunidades is aimed at rationalizing poor people's behaviors into responsibility and self-care. Its substructure *is* neoliberal. Cash transfer programs are not seen as welfare, where unconditional money is given to needy populations. Instead, the notion of conditionality restructures the population into a participating citizenry. The program is considered to move away from dependency altogether (Levy 2006) and toward the creation of active, engaged citizen-consumers.

A Particular Focus on Women

In many CCT programs, special emphasis is placed on women in a twofold manner: (1) the moment a girl begins her first year of secondary school, she begins to receive more money to discourage the high indices of drop-outs that begin at that grade; and (2) pregnant women receive particular attention to help the proper development of their pregnancy, to protect the mother's health, and to identify high-risk pregnancies (SEDESOL 2011). The central point of Oportunidades is that the beneficiary families are helped with the financial costs of having children in school (Molyneux 2006). Mothers are key to achieving these improvements in children's health and education. The primary aim of the program is to strengthen the mothers' responsibilities toward their children through workshops and monitoring.

Women are central to Oportunidades. Seeking to redress decades of programs that ignored the agentive potential of women, the women-in-development approach of Oportunidades sees the women as active agents of development rather than as passive and subordinate recipients of the government's largesse (Razavi and Miller 1995). Women's control of income has direct implications for family welfare. As Blumberg (1988) shows, where women have independent control of the family resources, they tend, more than men, to use them for their family and children's well-being. Such outcomes have additional implications for poverty alleviation programs. Browner and Leslie (1995) state that women are vital in maintaining the household economy as well as the health and well-being of their families.

However, Kate Bedford (2006) discusses why, from a feminist perspective, it is very problematic that women are seen as the "key" to development. She discusses how ostensibly women-centered programs may in fact be appropriating a language of women's empowerment to entrench a neoliberal agenda. Delving into the gendered approach in the World Bank, which advocates for greater female presence in the public sphere, and greater attention to men's loving nature in private spheres, she peels back the various contradictions that this can bring. This gendered approach encourages poor men to reduce their partner's reproductive and household burdens, thereby allowing the women to work outside the home. Bedford argues that this retains a very strong neoliberal core and is less about women's empowerment and gender equality than to socially engineer "loving, sharing partnerships" (2009:135). This becomes a cheap and expedient way to embed people into the market without having to invest much in social services. She states, "Gender and sexuality do not appear as distractions from serious critical debates about adapted neoliberalism." Instead, they form part of the very basis on which policymakers "engage with the new face of development, because inclusive neoliberalism involves a heightened reliance on policy formulations . . . to ensure the survival of the poor" (Bedford 2009:203).

In Amatlán, Adela was particularly happy with receiving Oportunidades money but was troubled by some of the disparities in the cash received. She stated,

> Here the girls can buy what they need for school, shoes, [their uniform]. [I tell them] not to spend it all. They want to use sanitary pads, [they need to pay for] school exams, [and] bus fare. [It is] 300 pesos for bus fare. . . . [Women] with many children [receive] much more money. Some [women] receive [money] for five children. Some said they received between 6,000 [and] 7,000 [pesos]. More children, more money. The government keeps us; the government supports us. The [girls] like to receive the money; they get happy when the support arrives. They must not squander it. I tell them to study, to work hard. They are being supported. Before there was no way to support one's self. . . . Some would want to study but they couldn't because they had no money.

When Adela's eldest son got a girl pregnant at the age of seventeen, the young family moved into Adela and her husband's household, as is traditional in this region. Her young daughter-in-law, only fifteen, would not be eligible for Oportunidades money, however, unless she established her own nuclear household—on her own plot of land. For Oportunidades, only the nuclear family arrangement counted. Many of the women in the village experienced this situation where their extended family structures were considered nuclear families for survey purposes. Blanca, a young mother who lived with her parents-in-law after marriage, said, "You only receive [money] if you live apart. As I live with my parents [-in-law] I don't receive it." Altagracia, who lived across from Esperanza, and whose daughter had moved back in with her young family while her husband worked as a policeman, said, "There are many [women] whose sons, whose daughters-in-law don't have Oportunidades." For these young mothers, the additional gendered protection from Oportunidades was not enough. By not being counted in the Oportunidades censuses, their mothering also did not count. Thus they slipped through the cracks created by an imperfect numerical system.

Becoming a Beneficiary

Families are enrolled in Oportunidades based on a marginality index determined through the national census data. Using this data, households across the country are ranked according to various factors and social indicators such as community marginality, population density, family income, and infrastructure, such as access to health and education facilities (Sridhar and Duffield 2006). Any household that falls below the poverty line is eligible for enrollment (Skoufias 2005).[24] For the first few years, only rural households were enrolled in Oportunidades, but since 2002, urban families are enrolled as well. The households determined to have the greatest need and those who were the most marginalized were the first families enrolled in the program.

The number of families enrolled by 2012 was 6.5 million, which is approximately 30 percent of all Mexican rural and urban households and almost 100 percent of those in extreme poverty (Inter-American Development Bank [IDB] 2003; SEDESOL 2012b). This is just over thirty-four million people. By 2012, in northern Veracruz, almost 850 thousand people were enrolled in the program (Instituto Mexicano del Seguro Social [IMSS] 2012), while in the municipality of Ixhuatlán de Madero, just under eight thousand five hundred families were enrolled (SEDESOL 2009), which is roughly 70 percent of families. In Amatlán, there were 103 enrolled families (SEDESOL 2009), which is 98 percent of the families in the village. The families that are not enrolled have alternative sources of income (such as commerce, transportation, or teaching) that push them slightly above the marginality index.

Because northern Veracruz is an area of extreme underdevelopment, the indigenous villages were some of the first ones enrolled in this program. As Esperanza told me one morning in 2004 as we sat in her home,

> Some people have been given the money from the beginning; that is six years. But not all [the women] were given from the beginning, first only some and then more signed up and requested [more Oportunidades] and then [the money] came to about twenty [more], and then they asked again and then about five [more received it] and little by little [everyone] was given. I was one of the first ones to receive [the money]; it has been six years. A lady came to take a census and many [women] were scared and did not want to open [the doors to their houses] for her, because they didn't know what she would ask them. I was not afraid. She came and I chatted with her. And then she says that she will ask me questions and I thought [to myself] "what am I going to answer?" but she would tell me [what to say]. She says, "Let's just put

that you have nothing," she tells me. And when she asks me how many cows I have and I am thinking what to answer, she says, "Let's just put that you just have only one," and that's what she did.

Esperanza's words demonstrate the Mexican state's interest in enrolling only the most marginalized—and those who "have nothing," as she narrates. It also shows two additional interesting aspects. One is the fact that only the women who opened the door to the interviewer were enrolled in the program. But in this region, and in many other indigenous areas, the most remote populations—and thus most marginalized—also tend to be the most reticent and wary of interacting with strangers. This poses a problem for enrollment: a woman becomes enrolled only if she is interviewed, but she might be interviewed only if she is not so marginalized and fearful of strangers. Second is the fact that the interviewer was keener to enroll as many women as possible than to obtain the most accurate census data. In Esperanza's case, it would have made little difference whether the truth or this bending of the truth was written down because she is very poor and thus would be a good candidate for enrollment. But it certainly opens up questions about data fabrication and whether some of the first enrollees were not as marginalized as the census indicated.

Impacting Health

There is no doubt that Oportunidades has had a markedly positive effect on the lives of its beneficiaries. The health of beneficiary women and children has increased with a simultaneous decrease in morbidity. The poorest and younger infants enrolled in the program have experienced an increase in height as well as a reduction in anemia (Rivera et al. 2004). Vulnerable populations receive nutritional supplements, in the form of a *papilla*—a pureed nutritional supplement—that has a full complement of necessary nutrients. Food consumption rates have also increased, which could also account for the increase in their caloric intake, and thus a decrease in anemia (Sridhar and Duffield 2006). Rivera et al.'s (2004) study of the effect of Oportunidades on children's growth and rates of anemia showed that the children who were enrolled in the program and who received nutritional supplements and whose mothers received nutritional education had better rates of growth and lower rates of anemia than children in comparable situations who were not enrolled in the program.

Much concern revolves around beneficiary families' diets. With illnesses such as diabetes and hypertension becoming common in rural areas, attention has been placed on informing mothers about the risks inherent in certain diets. Cristina recounted the information she had been given at the clinic: "Well, they say not too eat too much, only two or three tortillas. Not to eat until one is full. And then they say not to have coffee, nor soda, nor flavored water (like Kool-Aid), nor coffee when you eat bread. They take all that away. [They say] we should eat lots of vegetables. That's what the doctor says."

Yet even receiving Oportunidades money was not enough for some families to achieve better health. Juana put it thus: "If you have money, you get a treatment. If you don't have [money] you don't." Sridhar and Duffield (2006), in an evaluation of conditional cash transfers for Save the Children, also found that there was an increase in growth among enrolled children—who grew on average 1 cm more than nonenrolled children. They also found that there was an increase in immunization rates, as well as a 12 percent difference in illness among children under the age of five between children enrolled and not enrolled in Oportunidades. They attribute these changes to various factors, including access to primary health care, regularity of the transfers, *pláticas* attendance, and amount of the cash transfer.[25] The physician in Tepatepec acknowledged that vaccination had increased over time but that religious affiliation also played a significant role. He said, "There are many children in the other communities, less so in Amatlán. It is because those [communities] follow the Agua Viva [religion].[26] It gets quite difficult with them. They don't always want to follow things about health. Not all want to vaccinate."

Oportunidades has also had an impact on reproductive behavior. González Montes's (2008) data shows that, regarding family-planning education, 88.6 percent of the enrolled women (who ranged from twenty to forty-nine years of age) reported knowing at least one contraceptive method; this is slightly above nonbeneficiaries, 84.5 percent of whom were aware of contraceptives. Paz, who was concerned about keeping her family small, said, "There are almost no babies [in Amatlán]. In La Huerta there are lots. The women there do have children. There are lots of babies. But it's better with fewer children, as there is no money. Here the women *se cuidan* (take care not to get pregnant). There are many using the pill." Also significant in several evaluations of Oportunidades was that approximately 6 percent more beneficiaries than nonbeneficiaries were aware of methods such as the IUD and sterilization. González Montes also found that the most common contraceptive method among beneficiary women were sterilizations (around 45 percent of all contraceptive users) and the IUD (24.4 percent of beneficiaries who use contraceptives). Both these methods are the preferred forms of contraception promoted by the Mexican health and population sectors—primarily because they are semipermanent or completely permanent—and are the most widely offered by medical institutions. Thus once the women undergo these procedures, there is less follow up and worry that she will become pregnant. Also significant is the fact that 92 percent of women who used contraceptives obtained these methods from a medical institution. Prenatal care also increased with enrollment, with medical check-ups increasing from 84 to 89 percent. Although this increase might seem slight, for nonbeneficiaries the attendance rate was 84.4 percent in 1998 and 85.5 percent in 2000.

Skoufias (2005:22) argues that the impact on reproductive behavior is caused by an improvement of the "human capital embodied in children." According to him, this change possibly affects the number of children families would like to have. From the words of Estela that I included in the Introduction ("I am not family planning. After [my son] was born they put in the IUD over there in Poza Rica") emerges the curious notion that the phrase "to family plan" is a verb, and used by Estela as an active one at that. And so when an IUD is inserted, somehow a woman's agency is removed. The planning is done by the device instead of by her—putting into question notions of agency and empowerment for the beneficiary women. Skoufias points out that the monetary incentive provided by Oportunidades for families to invest in the education and health of their children is reinforcing alternatives to large numbers of children and that over time, the fertility and population growth in rural areas will be decreased.

Many of the women in Amatlán echoed this notion that fewer children were better, that there was more money to go around, and that it was easier with fewer children. Carole Browner and Joanne Leslie (1995) show that the hypothesis postulating an inverse relationship between women's work and income on the one hand and fertility behavior on the other is not nuanced enough, however. Indeed, they state that, while this hypothesis is generally supported in industrialized contexts, it is much more complex and variable in developing nations. They point out that one factor that might explain why women who have income or are part of the labor force might have many children is "the relative lack of conflict in developing countries between women's roles as workers and as mothers" (264). They add that this hypothesis is ethnocentric and does not apply to rural-based economies where women's work and child-care practices are frequently combined.

González Montes (2008) states that the incorporation of the nutritional supplements for infants aged newborn to two has not diminished the rate of breastfeeding. She found that, within her study, approximately 90 percent of women breastfed their children at least until nine months of age. My own data in Amatlán confirms this information, as the majority of women nursed their children from birth. Only 8.8 percent of the fifty-three women in my study did not breastfeed at all. Just under 3 percent of them breastfed less than a month. And slightly less than 90 percent breastfed for at least one year. Most of this latter group breastfed for significantly more than a year, with almost 12 percent of all the women nursing for over two years.

Yet there is a small—and problematic—caveat to add. All the young mothers with children under the age of two informed me that they were repeatedly told at the clinic that they had to wean their children as soon as they turned one year old. They were warned at the clinics that their milk "*ya no sirve*" (is no longer good) and that it was little better than water. My *comadre* Estela, whose young children in 2007 were three years and one year old respectively, anxiously confided in me that she was still nursing her infant boy. To repeat from this book's Introduction, she said, "The [doctor] says that we should stop breastfeeding at six months because [the milk] is spoiled, that it is only water and it is no longer good." She said she could not tell the staff at the clinic that she still breastfed because they always scolded her for nursing longer than necessary. Blanca echoed Estela's thoughts almost word for word when she verbalized her concerns with breastfeeding her one-year-old daughter, Célia:

> The nurses keep telling me not to give her [breast milk]. They say that my milk is no longer good; that now it is just water. [They] say it is better that I don't give her any more. When I have an appointment [at the clinic] I tell [Célia] not to ask me for *chichi* because if [she does] they scold me.[27]

The nurses stated that they encouraged complementary feeding after four months of age and the slow decrease of breast milk intake until the infant was weaned at one year. Concerned about the nutritional strength of breast milk, they argued that after one year it no longer had the necessary nutrients for toddlers and that mothers gave their children too much breast milk and not enough solid food. They emphasized that there was a direct and causal relationship between breastfeeding and local malnutrition. One of the nurses stated,

> [We encourage breastfeeding] until one year of age. [No more than that] because if we encourage breastfeeding until two to three years

the children usually become malnourished. Because the mother nurses the child and does not give it [solid] foods despite the fact that these should be given from four months onward; not just the milk. In the first four months only mother's milk. After the fourth month introduce solids. . . . But they don't do that; they just give it breast; it is just breast and breast. And the child at this stage, [well] breast milk doesn't have the necessary nutrients to help the baby develop. . . . If they are giving the baby a good diet and the child is nourished, if it is healthy, [and] with good weight they can continue giving it breast [milk] at a year, at two years. Yes, they can continue. But if the child is malnourished we tell the [mother] that it is better that she takes away the breast and she starts to offer it food. . . . There are some [mothers] who, for example, right now we have various malnourished children who will turn two years old and who are unable to increase their weight. Why? Because the mother insists 'he doesn't want to eat' and they just give it breast [milk]. And there the [children] waste their energies and on wasting energy they lose weight. And besides, they do not give them complementary feeding and when they want to [feed the child] then the child is already full. But it has grown full from that milk that, in my opinion, is just water that does not have the necessary nutrients to encourage [good health]. . . . I tell them, "you can give them the breast but only after having fed them." Because if they give them the breast first then the [child] will not want the food because it will already be full. The complementary foods should be given first and then give it the breast. . . . So, what does this mean? That there are some mothers who do not place enough importance on complementary nutrition.

This information is in direct contradiction to the precepts set by the World Health Organization, which encourages exclusive breastfeeding for six months and the continuation of breastfeeding alongside complementary foods until two years of age. Cecilia Van Hollen (2003) notes a similar situation among the women she worked with in India and the Baby Friendly Hospital they gave birth in. She shows how clinicians co-opted the development discourse of "traditional" and "backward" versus "scientific" to chide their patients into behaving according to modern expectations. She especially notes how it was the *knowledge* of the scientific underpinnings (and language) for feeding and child-care practices that was important in this discourse rather than the practices themselves.

What is problematic about the one-size-fits-all approach to child feeding at the clinics in Ixhuatlán is that either the women breastfeed covertly (and consequently they do not feel supported at the medical centers), or the women do indeed wean their children off breast milk but replace it with formula, or even worse—and of much more concern for infant health—with soft drinks. Over my years in Amatlán, I saw a fair share of toddlers running around their family homes carrying a baby bottle filled with cola drink, a behavior not unusual across Mexico and Latin America (Leatherman and Goodman 2005). None of the mothers saw this behavior as problematic, simply seeing soda as a prestigious product that was tasty, expensive, and desired, leading to what Leatherman and Goodman (2005) call the "coca-colonization" of the women's lives. Consequently, either of these behaviors—women breastfeeding against orders or giving their children soft drinks—runs into issues of compliance and their role as mothers. With both scenarios, they are perceived to be harming the health of their children through bad nutrition—it is the women's own bodies that fail them and let them down, and consequently, they let down their children and society at large.

Strengthening the Social Fabric: An Emphasis on Coresponsibility

The cash grants are attached to conditions regarding the health, education, and nutrition of the mothers and their children. As a condition of receiving the money, the mothers must make certain that their children attend government-run (mostly Spanish-language) school daily as well as go regularly to a medical center to receive nutritional and health care. The women are repeatedly told that the money they receive should be used for educating, clothing, feeding nutritious food to, and generally taking care of their children. The mothers are also expected to be involved in the medical centers as patients and participants.

Paz was a young mother in her early thirties whose son was almost twelve years older than her daughter. Her story was a sad one—she had lost her own mother to murder and her mother-in-law to kidney disease within the space of a couple of years. This made her feel very alone and out of place. She felt especially vulnerable when she had questions about mothering, often relying on her aunt Ofelia to guide her during moments of doubt. She depended heavily on Oportunidades:

> They give me 370 [pesos] and [they give] the boy 470 [pesos]. It is a little but it is enough for him to buy his shoes, his school things. . . . Well my husband and father-in-law work in the *milpa*. Almost no money is made that way; sometimes they'll sell the corn. They sell it in the market. So with the money from Oportunidades some money

comes in, but it is a little. . . . We have to go to the *pláticas* [instructional talks] in the clinic, go to the appointment at the clinic. If not they mark you as absent. Also one must do *faena* [work crew] at the *Casa* [*de Salud*] here. If not they mark them as absent. And also in the clinic. [One] has to go when one has an appointment, if not the doctor sees in the files that you have not gone and he reports you. And then those that have been reported don't receive more money.

Particular emphasis is placed on the "coresponsibility" of the enrolled families for their own development, where their active participation in the program's conditions is seen to overcome the historical welfarism and paternalism. Santiago Levy, one of the architects of Oportunidades, stated, "It really is money that people 'earn' by their good behavior . . . so families feel differently about [these] resources . . . to the extent that the mothers, in particular, feel that they've earned the right to these resources" (Public Radio International 2009).

The primary way that this program is seen to help eradicate extreme poverty is by strengthening women's position at home and in the community. This is achieved by making mothers the grantees of the program and the actual recipients of the cash transfers. Women, instead of men, are made the grantees because they are seen as more obedient (see Bedford 2009). As Doctor Braulio said, "The [people] are hard working. The women are much more responsible than the men. They do come to the check-ups and they bring their children. The men do not want to [come]. They [say] they have work or they are busy, but slowly but surely they are changing." It is this assumption about embodied responsibility that lies at the core of Oportunidades. Many mothers, in effect, become the economic heads of their household by virtue of having access to the transferred cash.

The coresponsibility and participation of the beneficiaries in their own development are what distinguish a cash transfer program from welfare, as the onus of (co-)responsibility for getting out of poverty falls on the recipient, not on the government. The Mexican government recognizes that social development will not be achieved solely through the government's intervention and that, instead, there must be a shared action that is based on social coresponsibility. This coresponsibility must be developed to "strengthen the social fabric [by] promoting participation and community development" (SEDESOL 2003:11, my translation). SEDESOL's *Citizen Manual* (2003), published to increase the transparency of various government assistance programs, emphasizes the several ways that women become an "active part in their own development, overcoming welfarism and paternalism" (29). They point out that children's attendance at school and families' attendance at the clinics "are the only condition(s) to remain in the Program" (29).

While the larger goal of the program is lofty, the coresponsibility is quite grounded and revolves primarily around meeting the conditions of the program. For instance, in order to receive the nutritional supplements, the "members of the beneficiary families must attend their medical appointments" and the titular beneficiary (the mother) must attend the "educational communication sessions" for health, nutrition, and hygiene (SEDESOL 2003:33, my translation), commonly known as *pláticas*. This neoliberal restructuring of people's behavior entailed their participation in a more active way in broader Mexico. Inés stated, "Well [even if I] don't want to go [to the clinic], when we have to we have to comply. There are a lot of people, the sun is strong, we have to line up, take a number."

Cristina eagerly awaited the monetary grants and was someone who took her coresponsibility very seriously. She stated, "With or without the support we always wanted to give the [children] an education. But it is better to receive the government's support." Gabriela, who did not receive Oportunidades because her son was yet too young and she lived in her parents-in-law's home, was disparaging of the cash grants, saying, "I don't like the idea of Oportunidades. I don't want my son to just receive money, instead he should learn to appreciate it and earn it." She said her husband agreed and that he thought the women demanded too much and that if they did not receive the money they complained. She added, "but they really shouldn't since the government owes them nothing."

Feeling indebted to the government, however, Cristina readily complied with the conditions, rationalizing it as follows: "We have to do it, [the government] has given us a very big support." Demonstrating how much she enjoyed participating, she rattled off all the things that she was expected to do.

> I like cleaning. You have to clean your *solar*, clean your home. And from cleanliness comes health. [We have to] boil water, help out our children more, put up a mosquito net during the rainy season because of the well-known dengue. They must not miss school; the teachers must work. Go to the clinic twice a year, and the little ones every two months for the first year. Have no pets in your home—dogs and chickens; be clean. The advantage of Oportunidades is that we can be hygienic, attend to our children, have good nutrition, . . . change our sheets, put up a mosquito net, put down a [concrete] floor. It is a very big support; it helps a lot. The *pláticas* help us a lot.

Oportunidades's aim is to tackle poverty by helping the poor population to "cope, mitigate, or reduce their risk of falling into or being trapped in poverty" (Molyneux 2006:433). It is based on the assumption that poor households do not invest sufficiently in their human capital and are thus caught in a cycle of poverty that is transmitted through the generations. According to Skoufias (2005), one of the first evaluators of the program, between 1997 and 1999 the program decreased poverty by 17 percent and the poverty gap by 36 percent in its beneficiaries. He ascribes the success of the program to the synergy caused by targeting nutrition, health, and education simultaneously as well as by moving away from food subsidies and instead empowering people through the use of conditional cash transfers.

The defining guidelines and vision of Oportunidades are focused on getting people out of poverty, especially placing great emphasis on the need for increased investing in girls so they are not taken out of school. While there are many problems with the implementation of the program, many advocates argue that it is necessary to do *something* to ensure that girls can be educated. The education of women has been argued to be one of the most important predictors for good health—including sexual and reproductive—for empowerment and for ameliorating poverty conditions that compel people to migrate in search of better options. Basu (2002) states, however, that while there is a correlation between education and empowerment, the mechanisms remain ambiguous. Indeed, the contributors to Jeffery and Basu's (1996) collected volume on education and fertility in South Asia show that even the assumptions about the connection between women's education, their autonomy, and their lower fertility are frequently ethnocentric and misguided. Educational achievement does not translate into more empowerment, as Alarcón-González and McKinley (1999) showed in their work on Mexico's structural adjustment period. They demonstrate how even though women's educational levels increased more than men's did during this time, overall they continued to earn much less.

The two Mexican economists who designed Oportunidades belong to the country's educational and economic elite and thus share many of the elite classes' racialized assumptions about poor and indigenous people. This is evident in their lack of problematizing the reasons that poverty and poor people exist to begin with or why so many poor people happen to be indigenous. Their ahistorical analysis does not ask why poor people also tend to be unhealthy and uneducated. They merely suggest that if nutritional, health, and educational advantages were made available to certain populations, then poverty would cease. Inherent within this model of development is surveillance—if no one is looking, then poor people will misbehave and engage in risky behaviors. Foucault (1995) would argue that making the poor population visible through a program like Oportunidades leads to power increasingly being asserted on the individual; these individuals can then be tracked and managed throughout their lives.

Oportunidades by itself—with its three-pronged focus on health, nutrition, and education—is just not enough. It is seen as a lifeline that will pull populations out of poverty. But without modifications to the socioeconomic or political landscape—that for most poor people is the ultimate cause of poverty—the issue will be unlikely to go away. How is Oportunidades restructuring gender relations at home? Will the women as the managers of large amounts of money actually have a voice in decision making with their partners? Will the mediocre (at best) education available in rural regions truly place these populations on a path to empowered citizenship? It is also troubling that in evaluating Oportunidades, the same factors that are conditional are the ones that are measured—and then held up as areas of accomplishment. If people are being given money to attend school, go to the clinic, and feed their children better, is it not reasonable to expect that the rates of school attendance would increase, that basic health would increase, and that people's access to nutritional supplements would also increase? Are these evaluations simply ascribing causation to the improvement rates of these factors, as opposed to reality—that it is simply correlational? Is there an independent evaluation of poverty eradication that would suggest that Oportunidades's strategy is working?

Oportunidades is in many ways simply a more materialized version of *indigenismo*. First, its primary tenets are to help indigenous populations (and poor rural and urban populations as well) to have better access to basic necessities, such as health, nutrition, and education. But the *form* that these services take mirror the mainstream Mexican ethos. Second, the primary aim is to encourage positive change in the behavior of the target population; they are expected to modify many of their current (obsolete or traditionalist) practices and adopt the (modern) ones deemed necessary to improve their lives. And third, the materializing comes from the use of the cash transfer. No longer is change toward modernity left to chance and occasional pressure from *mestizo* society; instead, a conditional cash transfer is used as both carrot and stick to—perhaps forcibly—achieve (or even coerce?) this modernity. I primarily see it as a neoliberal program that uses cash incentives to engineer citizen-consumers.

CHAPTER 2

From Eugenics to Parteras:

Changing Conceptions of Maternity

OPORTUNIDADES WAS CONCEIVED TO CREATE MODERN MOTHERS. USING this cash transfer program as a lens, we can analyze the ways that institutional forces impose a certain type of body politic on their subjects—particularly concerning reproduction. Linking the idea of disobedience with the broader perceptions of the women's reproduction can help to show connections between "good" motherhood and "good" citizenship. Oportunidades becomes a locus of modernity, with maternity and reproduction—and their control—becoming paramount at this locus. I focus on the idea of maternity in this chapter, rather than mothering, because maternity is the corporeal process of being pregnant, giving birth, and nurturing, through breast milk, the infant child (Jolly 1998). Additionally, as Jolly and others point out in the collected volume *Maternities and Modernities* (1998), mothers need to be relocated to the center of discussions about maternity—as they have historically been marginalized from these discussions. Within modernity and reproduction, women's bodies are modified through modern family-planning techniques, and most importantly, they can be counted among the numbers of a modern nation (Van Hollen 2003).

Contextualizing Mexican Modernity: Eugenics Lends a Hand

Mexico's health and education sectors have an interesting history firmly rooted in visions of modernization. During the exceptionally devastating and destructive revolution, the country lost almost 5 percent of its population—through outright violence, epidemics, and migration to the north. Aftereffects of the war were also felt in the extremely high infant mortality rate of over 20 percent. A prominent cause of the high infant mortality rate was the absence or scarcity of potable water and the destruction of the sewage systems during the violence. The Mexican state responded to this devastation and death by making an effort to become progressive and modern and by rebuilding the country's infrastructure—building and developing banks, roads, radiotelegraphy, dams, irrigation, and industry (Stern 1999). The state was especially concerned with the connection between progress, individual responsibility, and collective welfare (Bliss 2002).

According to feminist scholar Mary Kay Vaughn (2000), the intent of these early development policies was to bring order to the household and subordinate it to the interests of the nation's growth. In order to carry out this subordination, the process of rationalizing domesticity (Vaughn 2000:196) began to take place. Throughout most of the colonial and postcolonial periods in Mexico (and, indeed, the world), men existed in the public domain while women existed in the private, domestic domain. While this structure did not change much after the Mexican Revolution in the early twentieth century, the state sought to rationalize this division between public and private, men and women. The production of citizens to help develop the state became a paramount ideology, and mothers were perceived to be the key to citizen creation. Thus women—especially mothers—had to be educated "for scientific, hygienic household management and child raising in order to produce healthy, efficient, patriotic citizen-workers" (Vaughn 2000:196).

To fully grasp the ideology of building the modern nation-state present in Mexico in the early twentieth century, and to understand how modern Mexico's belief system concerning development emerges from its past, we need to explore the role the eugenics movement played in shaping the Mexican welfare state. While the Mexican Eugenics Society gained many of its ideas from American and European eugenic ideologies, it also took a uniquely Mexican turn. Eschewing the nature versus nurture debate, Mexican eugenicists firmly stood by the idea of environmental determinism (Stern 1999). As opposed to eugenicists elsewhere, where the problems of society were linked to the degeneration of the races through admixture, Mexican politicians, scholars, educators, and artists took up the idea of *mestizaje*—racial (and cultural) mixing (with "superior races")—as their platform for creating a new population, guided by women's reproduction.[1] And while the term eugenics can conjure up images of Nazi Germany and the idea of a master race, the eugenics present in Mexico during the early twentieth century did not follow that path. On the contrary, it was embraced by people who fought for the downtrodden and "*los de abajo*," the underdogs—a term memorialized by Mariano Azuela (2008) in his eponymous novel about the Mexican Revolution—and by those who thought that biological and social betterment would result in an improved citizenry.

For Mexican policy makers, the ills of the society were linked to structural and class-based—that is, environmental—issues beyond the ills of the social body. According to them, the Mexican lower class were sick and weak because of a rapacious system of landlords and priests and an unjust distribution of property and wealth (Vaughn 2000). Such a system was perceived to naturally result in (stereotypical) behaviors—men being macho men and women being submissive—that were troubling to the state as they led to unmodern populations. Such stereotypical behaviors were increasingly correlated with the problems of the state—unemployment, lack of citizen action, and too many "unwanted" Mexicans (Laveaga 2007).

Interested in recrafting the emerging Mexican state to compete on the world stage with developed and "advanced" nations, Mexican eugenicists focused on issues surrounding reproduction and socialization to create a strong citizenry with good genetic—and behavioral—characteristics. Motherhood came under scrutiny "as an object of knowledge and target of intervention" (Molyneux 2000:49). Motherhood was brought into discourses of national duty—to be mindful about women's provision of the next generation as maternity and fertility became "crucial resources for the nation justifying state regulation of women's bodies" (Molyneux 2000:50). Women bore the larger burden of maintaining domestic health because they gave life to the next generation. As Stern (1999:375) shows in her work on the history of the eugenics movement in early modern Mexico, "the health of babies was placed upon mothers, whose rearing practices were increasingly monitored and tied to the nation's need to secure a vigorous and healthy descent." Women were counseled in "responsible motherhood" (Stern 1999:375) to achieve these goals. This intervention frequently took the form of encouraging women not to become pregnant, or even sterilizing those who were seen as biologically and socially defective.

Feminist eugenicists were concerned with the effect that socially degenerative ills would have on women within the male-dominated society. Interestingly, their concerns in many ways mirror our present-day anthropological concerns with structural violence, wherein the women might be ill-equipped to find well-paying jobs and are exposed to sexual and domestic violence; both of these factors make the women vulnerable to poverty. Moreover, such a situation might cause the women to resort to certain activities—prostitution or alcoholism—that either generate income or are coping mechanisms. The feminist eugenicists were concerned with these populations as they were the next generation of mothers, and the health and hygiene of their children—and the collective—lay in the balance. In this paradigm, the individual mother bore the responsibility for the collective welfare (Bliss 2002). Mothers thus gave birth not only to their children but to the nation as well.

The idea of targeting motherhood as part of a civilizing and racialized modernizing mission has a long, global history (see Hunt 1988; Jolly 1998; Manderson 1998; Boddy 2007). That is, the domestic sphere, *in particular*, is usually the target for these kinds of civilizing projects. Emulating countries in Europe that were also recrafting their maternity welfare approaches as national duties, rather than just moral ones (Hunt 1988), Mexico specifically focused on maternity, sexuality, and children. Each of these factors was perceived to be a node of influence on the capabilities of the citizenry. Using the mutual processes of "cultural incorporation and transformation" (Hunt 1990:449), development and modernizing efforts were particularly successful. Of particular note is the fact that the conjoining of maternity with modernity is not just a revisiting of the traditional role of women as the primary caregivers, but is also a strong "rearticulation of all points of power within the domestic domain" (Stern 1999:371–72). And it is only through such a connection that modern citizens could be created while existing ones were reshaped.

One of the core beliefs at the time was in the neo-Lamarckian theory of inherited acquired characteristics, where an effort was made to produce a maternal body untainted by unclean and unsanitary behaviors—such as disease or inappropriate sexual unions.[2] To this end, the state focused on puericulture (an ideology to scientifically cultivate children) and a pronatalism tempered by biological selection and fitness (Stern 1999).[3] To develop puericulture, women's domesticity was to be rationalized and hygienicized. Mothers in households were the primary targets: new "scientific" discourses of human development, hygiene, nutrition, and health were disseminated to mothers from problematic backgrounds; mothers were to learn proper ways of providing nutritious food to their children; traditional birth attendants were discouraged; inoculations were of paramount importance; and sanitation changes (adding latrines, burning garbage, boiling water, removing stagnant water, and so forth) were expected.

Puericulture remains embedded within Mexican policies. Oportunidades is a perfect example of this melding of biological citizenship and cultural belonging. As in other spaces where global North and global South have in-

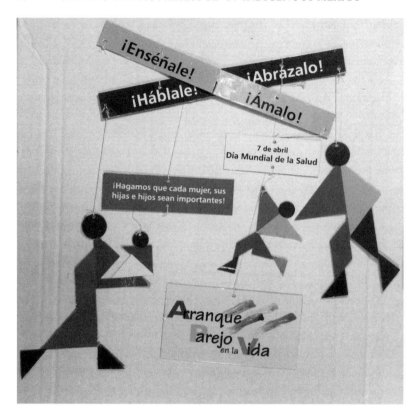

Figure 2.1. Arranque Parejo en la Vida mobile

tersected, mothers have been targets of efforts to civilize the citizenry. Boddy (2007) notes British efforts in colonial Sudan intent on civilizing the domestic and reproductive lives of women. Hunt (1990) describes the efforts of the Belgian colonists in Congo, who focused their attention on the *foyer social*—the social homes—that were domestic training homes for African women living in urban areas. In these social homes, gender roles, domestic space, and family life were revised and refashioned so women could represent moral standards through the "'civilized' institution of the nuclear family" (Hunt 1990:451). By making mothers the main target, such "civilizing" policies can be injected into the core of the family structure. In this way, the socialization of the new Mexican citizens begins at home, and the children become increasingly Mexicanized and integrated into the *mestizo* lifestyle.

One of the workers at the clinic in Ixhuatlán, Manuel, said very proudly one day, "We are not here to change [women's] customs; we simply come to tell them how they are wrong." Manuel works as a health liaison between Oportunidades and the enrolled women. He organized *pláticas*—informative talks—to impart information to the women and encourage them to modify their mothering practices. In his office hung a mobile designed by the Arranque Parejo en la Vida program (An Equal Start to Life), whose mission was to decrease maternal and infant mortality nationwide.[4] Manuel's mobile had some of the key concepts and phrases used by the program. With imperative phrases—such as "Love your child!" "Teach your child!" and "Breastfeed your child!"—it was designed to instill certain important health and hygiene values in women to encourage them to be good mothers (see figure 2.1).

Manuel's statement above epitomizes the state's belief in the erroneous nature of indigenous practices; it also shows how the practices to be eliminated are those that the government considers to be obstacles to progress and modernity. Women are expected to adopt the mainstream *mestizo* practices to become modern. The women's motherhood and mothering are in question, to be replaced by the modern, advanced, and scientific ideas of the Mexican state. Thus in one fell swoop, the women's indigenousness and their maternity can be reconceived to fall in line with the correct forms of identity.

Oftentimes development programs of the size of Oportunidades are linked to structural adjustment. Oportunidades is not a structural adjustment program in the strict sense of the word, as the funding is aimed at implementing social programs rather than at opening up the market or developing industry. It could be argued, however, that for the enrolled women it *does* imply structural adjustment, as the money is conditional on certain behavioral adjustments that will build human capital—and improve the workforce—for the country. Ultimately, conditional cash transfers center on changing risky and problematic behaviors in the population. One can even consider Oportunidades to have Lamarckian tendencies whereby, through puericulture and rationalizing domesticity, mothers will be able to transfer good citizenship and modernity to their children, who in turn will become better citizens and pass on these characteristics to subsequent generations. Cynthia Mahmood (1993) noted a similar development situation in India, where Adivasi (indigenous) girls were brought into boarding schools to be resocialized as "modern." The premise was that once they became mothers they would enculturate their own children into the modern values preferred by the state. Mahmood's example, and in many respects Oportunidades, are what Michael Hechter (1999) would call "internal colonialism" where peripheral populations lose the privilege of determining their own fate.

Gabriela Laveaga (2007) provides a historical analysis of the use of social structures, such as soap operas and slogans, to transform people's reproductive patterns in Mexico. She tracks several books and pamphlets written
between the 1940s and the 1960s that show the stratified reproduction
embedded within Mexican ethos. One of the books, written by a physician, shows several drawings of economically disadvantaged populations
and the number of children they have. Upon accessing the book myself, I
observed one of the images she referred to, which shows a woman kneeling
on a sidewalk against a tumbled-down wall; she has two children clinging
to her. One of them is in a *rebozo*—a sling—and is obviously a baby.[5] The
caption reads, "With such modest means is it right for them to have so
many children?" As Laveaga notes, the term *them* is particularly vague, and
could mean anything from women to indigent, or, most likely, indigenous
people. What perhaps is most surprising is that the woman only has two
children, not the "so many" indicated by the caption, which leaves one to
ponder whether "these people" were allowed to reproduce at all.

This mindset does not just belong to physicians in the 1960s or to urban dwellers. Indeed, one of the physicians I spoke with adamantly stated,

> "The woman from the countryside is very fertile, she has a lot of
> children. If you take away their [hormonal] contraceptive, by the
> next month they are already pregnant. Not so in the city. There the
> women take even six months for the body to get rid of the toxins. But
> here they get pregnant right away."

A nurse I spoke to at the same time blamed the women's behavior and
practices, stating, "It's because they do not practice the *cuarenteno* [the
forty-day rest period recommended by Mexican physicians] postpartum,
that is why." These convictions reflect what Laveaga (2007:29) refers to
as the transformation of the family-planning argument from "a scientific
one (the use of hormones to alter biology) to a socially responsible one"
whereby the state "pressure[s] the poor and socially undesirable under the
all-embracing rubric of population control." Through this policy, the state
aimed to forge a better society not only by creating better citizens but also
by having fewer of them (Laveaga 2007:30). Pregnancies should thus be
willed—women should individually control and space their births, and a
collective body (society, the state, and so on) needs to know what populations are having how many children (Ruhl 2002:643). Such an ideology
places responsibility and blame squarely on women—and mothers—and

even goes so far as to blame the ecological crisis on "overly fertile women"— as the physician does in Amatlán.

The corollary to the above concern is, of course, the concern of the physicians who treat the indigenous communities have over their individual patients' health and well-being. Perhaps the main issue is that physicians fail to see some of the cultural and historical causes for the high fertility rate. The language of their arguments and cajoles have two targets: either they point to the men—seen as *machos* who dominate and abuse their women— or they point to how having fewer children would immeasurably improve the women's lives and give them financial solvency. Doctora Felipa's concerns with the health of her female patients exemplify this idea:

> We have to tell this person the advantages of the operation, the physical benefit that it can have, the economic benefit. Because if she has many kids logically she will have more problems in supporting her family [and] giving primacy to education. So I tell them, "look, it's just that if you have four kids, who lives better? The [woman] who has four kids or the one who has two? Who looks younger? Mrs. So-and-so who has had an operation, or the other Mrs. So-and-so who has not been operated and has six kids, right?" So I make certain parallels so that they can see that it is better to be operated and have a more tranquil life, without risk of becoming pregnant, and that she is physically better off than someone who has so many kids and will keep on having [them]. Additionally if they are older women, the risk they can have [is great]. Because I tell them, "look, your husband can find another woman, but your kids will not get another mother. . . .' So in that way I start to make them aware and I give them guidance, which is why I have so many women who are waiting for the next [sterilization] campaign."

These arguments fit squarely into the Mexican ethos of recrafting the population and doing away with "backward" behaviors—such as machismo in men and submissiveness in women (Laveaga 2007). Moreover, Felipa expresses a particularly middle-class sentiment, which in turn emphasizes the populations' behaving like the middle-class—having fewer children and placing primacy on education. But such a belief puts the cart before the horse: the women will not become middle-class by having fewer children; instead, women who have small families do so *because* they are middle-class (see Jeffery and Basu 1996). Her arguments become effective, not so much because of the promise of living better and more fulfilled lives as women, but because of the fear of losing their lives and leaving their children motherless.

Voluntary Motherhood: Feminist Historical Context for Oportunidades

Politics in Mexico has historically been a male enterprise. Ortiz-Ortega and Barquet (2010), two female Mexican social scientists, point out that over the past forty years, Mexican women have worked collectively to construct a voice for various expressions beyond traditional ideas of citizenship, such as "bodily integrity, violence against women, the sexual division of labor, and the recognition of diverse expressions of sexualities" (108). Feminists in the 1960s began to address the specifics of their own social standing in the country, focusing especially on issues of reproduction, abortion, and motherhood. These feminists coined the term "voluntary motherhood" to refer to their demands to have control over their reproductive lives (Ortiz-Ortega and Barquet 2010)—these demands included abortion rights, comprehensive sexuality education, and eradication of forced sterilizations (Billings et al. 2002; Lamas 1997). This feminist critique became the legal antecedent for Mexico's legalization of contraception in 1974 (Ortiz-Ortega and Barquet 2010).

Former president Luis Echeverría, in 1974, enacted and amended several laws to establish the principle of equality between men and women. He even established a group within CONAPO, formed by academics, policymakers, and clergy, to discuss abortion. While the group recommended that abortion be decriminalized and be offered as part of health services, this recommendation never saw the light of day (Lamas 1997). Lamas (1997) points out that Mexico continues to reject economic reasons for abortion yet accepts eugenic and health reasons for it (such as HIV-related reasons). Nonetheless, there were many changes to the status of women in society. Ortiz-Ortega and Barquet (2010) note three distinct reactions to these changes by women: conservative women were indignant because these laws did not reflect their realities; liberal women close to government circles were in approval; and members of the nascent feminist movement expressed outrage that the government was "imposing a woman's agenda without women's participation" (114).

The following year, Mexico hosted the UN's First International Conference on Women. At this juncture is where ideas from women-in-development (WID) began to be incorporated actively into policy and development programs (Razavi and Miller 1995). This meeting had three primary objectives: (1) Full gender equality and the elimination of gender discrimination; (2) the integration and full participation of women in development; and (3) an increased contribution by women toward strengthening world peace (UN 2011). It especially urged governments to frame national strategies, targets, and priorities for achieving these goals. This conference effectively shifted focus from demography and population control to women's rights in the context of sexual and reproductive rights. In Mexico, women's legal status benefitted, including the abolishment of certain discriminatory labor laws and increased access of women to ownership of agrarian land (Ortiz-Ortega and Barquet 2010). Yet abortion continued to be illegal, and as Ortiz-Ortega and Barquet (2010:115) point out, "The legality of contraception but the illegality of abortion was a metaphor of women's conditioned access to the public arena; they gained access only through others' representations of their demands."[6]

By the mid-1990s, and on the heels of the 1995 Beijing UN International Conference on Women and the UN's International Conference on Population and Development (ICPD), held in Cairo in 1994, women and reproductive health and family planning were suddenly thrust into the spotlight and into policy makers' agendas. The discourse of sexual and reproductive health and rights and voluntary motherhood, among other concepts, has permeated programs and policies (at least on paper) since the mid-1990s. And ideas that had traditionally belonged solely to feminist activists were becoming part of everyday discourse (Lamas 1997). The Zapatista uprising in 1994 also gave voice to some of the concerns that indigenous women had regarding gender relations. These women "expanded the concept of democracy as they searched to root it in their different and traditional spaces—the home, the family, their community, and society in general" (Ortiz-Ortega and Barquet 2010:125).

In 1995, after the ICPD, Mexico redesigned its health services to reflect some of the conference's recommendations. The General Directorate of Reproductive Health was created, which included the Department of Gender and Development (Rosenbaum 1995). This directorate merged the older directorates of maternal and child health and of family-planning services under one umbrella ministry. The primary goals of its overall gendered perspective were to provide family planning, adolescents' reproductive health care, women's health care, and safe motherhood, and to prevent sexually transmitted diseases. Paola Sesia (2007), an anthropologist working in the state of Oaxaca in Mexico, notes that there are several shortcomings to this gendered perspective—namely that only women (and not men) are included for reproductive health services and family planning, and that much of the wording of the new directorate was vague about reproductive "rights," leading to a considerable gap between discourse and practice.

A Focus on Women's Empowerment

The term empowerment has been used in development since the 1980s and is generally understood as a "process of transformation involving both the acquisition of capabilities and changes in subjectivity that enable agency to be exercised" (Molyneux 2006:429). It is not only the ability to make choices (that is, agency), but also being able to shape what choices are available. It tends to take a "bottom-up" approach to changing gender power relations, to making these populations aware, and to building their capacity to challenge status quo (Reeves and Baden 2000). Empowerment is linked to the concept of participation. The reasoning is that when poor and marginalized people become empowered, they gain more voice in decision-making arenas and also develop the capabilities that enable them to escape poverty (see Laveaga 2007). These populations thus move away from being "welfare cases" or "beneficiaries" of the state and instead are seen as becoming agents who are capable of recognizing their own needs and engaging in the setting of priorities.

Empowerment models have focused on a variety of factors to involve people in agency creation. Literacy programs are one such way to increase local participation in larger processes, thus leading to the participants' empowerment. Ghose (2001) argues that education is never neutral (especially across cultures) and that even literacy programs need to explicitly try to change power relations at a social and individual level. In her work in a literacy program in northern India, she shows that for women to feel empowered as a result of an engagement with education, they must be empowered within the educational practice. Literacy is a skill that enables women to deal with their environment from a position of strength. The women in Ghose's study demanded literacy to redefine their changing realities—including developing new skills, interacting with power structures, having greater mobility and self-confidence, and desiring information on a range of issues. Projects such as these follow the ideas of Paulo Freire, who argued that literacy itself is not an empowering tool but it is the *type* of literacy that can empower people. He pushed for the development of local literacies to develop *concientizaçao* ("conscientization") and for people to use literacy "for personal and social enlightenment, to reflect on their experience, and to see themselves as agents in their own lives rather than passively accepting the roles assigned to them by others" (Olson and Torrance 2001:7). Thus Freire advocated for literacy in reading land rights documents, development policies, and government materials, and in other areas that would lead not only to a literate population but also to one that was politically savvy—and empowered.

Beneficiary women are expected to be empowered through their enrollment in Oportunidades and through their compliance with the conditions—especially coresponsibility and self-care. Their empowerment is meant to be reflected in their choices about their reproductive bodies— having control over the number and spacing of children, their birth choice, and their eventual child-care practices. However, women's compliance with Oportunidades is monitored by both teachers and clinicians. Any noncompliance with the conditions may result in removal from the program. This results in a significant disempowerment over their bodies. Adela stated in regard to certain women's noncompliance, "They will report them and they will take away the support from Oportunidades." Hence many of the women frequently went to great lengths to attend the *pláticas* and their medical appointments. Emma, Jacqueline's mother, said one day,

> [We have to go to the clinic today] because they want to have a *plática*. But if we don't go they tell us they will take away our support, our [Oportunidades money]. But the doctor doesn't even come all the way over here [although he has a car]. No, we all have to go over there, but it is not easy because the children come [home] from school and the men come back [from the fields] and they have to be fed and then the women are not around.

One of the teachers, Aurora, who lives in the village and prides herself on being very politically savvy (and who does not receive Oportunidades money because she does not fall within the marginality index), thought that the women needed to be more assertive at the clinic. She said,

> I tell these women that they should not be pushovers at the clinic. And they give the *pláticas* to the women and what I tell them is that it would be better if the doctor and nurse came here, since here we have the *Casa de Salud* and that's what it is for.[7] But the doctor doesn't come. But when I tell the women they say 'no, that one should not

[complain]' and so off they go. There are some who cannot [walk] well, others carry their children, but there they go. . . .

Adela's, Aurora's, and Emma's words encourage one to question just how empowering women's enrollment in Oportunidades really is. Gloria expressed some dissatisfaction with the program, particularly the system of reports and black marks that would affect her enrollment. Mentioning that she often missed appointments at the clinic because of the amount of work she had at home, she said, "But I don't miss willingly." She added that she missed appointments much more when her twin girls were younger "because I could not leave them." She said because of this, "I was always marked as absent and was constantly reported. I would lose my money for a while. Now I can go more often because the kids are older. They do scold at the clinic. I don't like it. They always tell me to have an operation." From her words it is evident that she did not feel empowered by participating in the conditions. Indeed, she chose the management of her household and of her children over compliance with the monetary conditions and being treated as an errant child.

Oportunidades's secondary outcomes of building the mothers' capacities, empowerment, and citizen participation, as well as strengthening community ties and gender equality, are invisible. Most of the emphasis lies in the effects on the triad of health, nutrition, and education. The actual implementation and measurement of these secondary outcomes remains nebulous at best, as the interpretations regarding them have varied over time and the "quality of what is on offer under these headings depends upon local authorities and cooperating professionals" (Molyneux 2006:434). Additionally, by naturalizing women's roles as mothers and by making their enrollment indirectly contingent on compliant maternity, these policies are in effect disempowering the women. Paradoxically, while the women are expected to be good mothers (and providers), they have to cut into their household and child-care duties in order to receive the money. Ultimately their roles as wives and mothers can suffer. How then are the women empowered?

The notions of empowerment and coresponsibility within Oportunidades are not necessarily about developing individual agency but have come to mean that poor people are to be trained and educated to prepare them for employment (Molyneux 2006). Thus Gabriela's words mentioned earlier perfectly illustrate this conflict, as she saw a dependence on the government as disempowering, while her own actions of finding a job as a maid or accompanying her husband in his work as a tinker gave her the status and income she desired.

Cornwall and Brock (2005:1045) level a particularly lively critique at the "buzzwords" used in the development schemes of the past couple of decades—specifically "empowerment," "participation," and "poverty reduction." They state,

> Many of the familiar terms of recent years evoke a comforting mutuality, a warm and reassuring consensus, ringing with the satisfaction of everyone pulling together to pursue a set of common goals for the well-being of all. Participation, poverty reduction and empowerment epitomise this feel-good character: they connote warm and nice things, conferring on their users that goodness and rightness that development agencies need to assert the legitimacy to intervene in the lives of others.

They specifically state that these words, emerging from deep, complex histories evoking civil rights, self-help philosophies, or feminist scholarship, have been rendered apolitical in the one-size-fits-all approach to development. They state that the words are mostly used with a neoliberal agenda of accountability, governance, and partnership—which do not evoke the "warm and nice things" that they are intended to evoke.

Despite its self-proclaimed gendered and empowering approach, Oportunidades has failed to tackle the underlying causes of gender inequality in Mexico. Indeed, there is much feminist literature (Bedford 2009; Karim 2008) that would argue that it is precisely this gendered approach that causes inequality to be entrenched. Molyneux (2006) states that it is solely through the recognition of their children's needs that the mothers receive the cash transfers, in order to better fulfill their maternal responsibilities. As in the many social and welfare programs that have historically been developed in Latin America, these social policies are not gender-blind but rather function with gendered conceptions of social needs, which are familial, patriarchal, and paternalistic. So even though girls gain access to education and health, and many have entered the workforce, their mothers (who also form a large part of the workforce) have their family, as opposed to their own empowerment, as their primary duty. The mothers in many ways have become expendable in the drive to create modern citizens—they are literally and figuratively the vessels used to carry and bring children up into modern Mexican life. And though economists such as Wodon et al. (2003) point out that Oportunidades has created an increase in girls' enrollment in secondary school, perhaps their education comes at the expense of their mothers' empowerment and control over their bodies and lives.[8] It will not be until the subsequent generation of women that we are likely to see an improvement of these girls' future status in their households and any long-term empowering effect on them.

Concern about women's empowerment through obedience to the accepted national norms of family planning is also present among the clinicians. Doctora Felipa at the Ixhuatlán clinic summed it up when she said, "But on the whole, well, I think [the women] have become more *concientizadas*, and we have quite a few patients family planning." Her use of the word *concientizada*—so similar in form to Freire's *concientizaçao*—is interesting. As in Portuguese, this Spanish term implies that a person has agency in decision making, wherein they have eschewed passivity and instead taken control over their (reproductive) life. Yet there is also an implication of obedience in this word, where somehow a person who is *concientizada* is following the larger rules of society. The way it is used in Mexico assumes that prior to being *concientizada*, the person was either willfully ignorant or irretrievably stupid. Thus within this same definition there is a duality of agentive and passive (or compliant) action.

If this is how we define empowerment—as a means to become agents who are engaged and involved in larger processes—then Oportunidades seems to fall short. While it includes the coresponsibility of the women in their own development, much of this is about developing the capacities of their children. There is no overt effort within Oportunidades to empower the women as actual agents—whether through literacy efforts or Freire's *concientizaçao*. Though the program involves women in the physical development of their children, and that of their families, the women continue to exist within a patriarchal system that tells them what to do and expects them to behave in the proper maternal way. The program conserves the traditional division of labor, where women are the primary caretakers of their children's health and well-being (González-Montes 2008; see also Clark 1993). They are also held responsible for the health of the community.

Compliance is expected from the enrolled women; this compliance goes beyond simply "behaving cooperatively" in the clinic and also includes participating in any events, requirements, and expectations of the clinic-Oportunidades dyad. Such expectations included attending *pláticas*, visiting the clinic, following medical orders, and even cleaning the clinic and its surroundings. This last was a particularly curious expectation, as it emphasized the communal aspect of the clinic—where all people are participants and should contribute to its existence—while simultaneously stipulating that it was the clinicians who were in charge of the clinic and any women who did not contribute to its upkeep would be sanctioned by the staff. The required act of sweeping the *Casa de Salud* or the clinic before a *plática* was seen by the women as both necessary and participatory. Though the women I spoke with tended to unquestioningly participate in the cleaning activities, it was often a burdensome task to travel to the clinic at the expense of their domestic duties.

Lamia Karim (2008) has written a profound critique of development programs that include a gender component. Focusing on Bangladesh's microcredit programs, she illustrates the way that women are sacrificed for the greater good. Focusing on what she calls the "economy of shame"—whereby modern institutions (such as microcredit programs) have co-opted the use of public shaming—she shows how it has become an effective means of social control over the grantee women. These women are consequently held responsible for the sanctity of their families' honor. Additionally, she shows how women, while the carriers of the loans, were almost never the end users of the money; instead their husbands and male relatives used it. While this gender structure is not unusual across the world, what Karim is especially critical of is the suppression of this information by the development programs. Such silencing means that development programs and NGOs can theoretically check the box for their inclusion of women in development. More troubling, however, is that women are especially sought out as subjects for development because they are seen as more docile and more manipulable to the needs of the state. This system allows for a profound entrenchment of power relations. In the end, as I also show in my work among the Amatlán women with Oportunidades, the women's rights are sacrificed—and the women themselves are expected to be self-sacrificing—to the greater human capital development of their children, and ultimately the country.

"Making them aware": Creating a Reproductive Habitus

All these forces and institutions—from development, to the state and nation-state, to whether one is indigenous or Mexican, have all framed and shaped Mexican women's model for maternity and reproduction. The confluence of these historical, processual, and structural factors resonates with the global system, where inequities become part and parcel of women's embodied experiences of reproduction. Building upon Miller and Shriver's (2012) work on women's habitus, preferences, and birth choices, and upon Cartwright's (2008) habitus of motherhood, I propose the reproductive habitus as a frame of analysis. This model allows one to contextualize the women's reproductive bodies and interactions. By understanding their habitus, the gray area between themselves and the institutions that shape them, we can gain more definition. This approach links the larger structures of power to the intimate ways the women live in their bodies. The reason that I have focused on the reproductive habitus of a marginalized population is that their lives more sharply feel the constant give-and-take between their daily actions and their formation and definition by broader processes.

Much of the emphasis on women's bodies lies in what I refer to as their biopotentiality—their ability to turn the products of their bodies into potential citizens for the nation. Biopotentiality is a term I have refashioned from biology that originally referred to the potential of a tissue to develop into different structures. I have transformed this word into one that has broader application to the ways that bodies interact with themselves, those around them, and larger societal expectations. The philosopher Roberto Esposito briefly used this term in his analysis of Nietzsche, stating, "No politics exists other than that *of* bodies, conducted *on* bodies, *through* bodies" (Esposito 2008:84, emphasis in original). It is thus by analyzing the micropractices of the women's bodies that we can understand the ways women live in them and how they are shaped for the ultimate production of future generations.

I additionally draw from Marcel Mauss's (1973) techniques of the body, Pierre Bourdieu's (1977) embodiment of dispositions and habitus, and Mary Douglas's (1986) analysis of how institutions structure people's decisions to create the concept of reproductive habitus. Moreover, I use Oka and Fuentes's (2010) idea of niche construction to examine how people modify the functional relationship between themselves and their (social) environment.

Habitus is a theoretical concept that explains how a person's structural and class position becomes embodied as unconscious dispositions—which are expressed in basically anything a person may do, from one's posture and gestures, to how one walks, eats, sleeps, and awakens (Mauss 1973), to how one combs one's hair or blows one's nose. Habitus is processual, existing in the hazy gray realm between consciousness and unconsciousness. Margaret Lock (1993:137) refers to habitus as a "repetition of unconscious, mundane bodily practices." In *Intimate Apartheid* (2007), Bourgois and

Schonberg explore the "ethnicized habitus" that is reinforced through daily interaction among homeless heroin addicts. Divisions based on skin color are embodied in the addicts' techniques of the body through their choice of injection site. Bourgois and Schonberg use Mauss to show how many of these techniques are preconscious. Specifically, the practices carry symbolic power implications and are naturalized as deficiencies or superiorities. Dispositions shape how one sees the world and how one reacts to it.

An important aspect of habitus is that it is an embodiment of institutions. Additionally, a person's habitus is dependent on history and memory; members of a social group frequently share habitus as they share a collective history and they exist within a particular social, political, economic, and natural environment that continually shapes their habitus. People respond to this environment and unconsciously develop their habitus, yet they also in turn—through their responses to stimuli—will shape their environment and the institutions. This is where niche construction comes in.

The idea of niche construction used by Oka and Fuentes is primarily ecological and evolutionary in scope—looking at the effect of predatory pressure and of cooperation on human selection and evolution. I suggest that niche construction can also occur with a person or population's social, economic, and political environments. The predatory pressure in this case would be the pressure from institutions and larger society. Lest it be thought that predation is too harsh a word to describe institutional pressure, Oka and Fuentes define it as "an external force that causes the attrition of individuals, resources, and labor within a group" (2010:8). It is especially the larger coercive pressure from the elite classes or other powerful institutions that curtail segments of people's activities with the forcible embedding of the people's lives within the larger Mexican state. Within a state, where institutions and bureaucracy are the norm, the big decisions are made by the state, leaving the small decisions to us (Douglas 1986). Decisions are made at the interface between individual action and institutional structure; but that very structure also affects individual action.

The women of Amatlán's reproductive habitus is a complex of behaviors regarding reproductive and sexual practices, contraceptive choices, childcare practices, and mothering practices. And while each individual woman has her own habitus, there are many behaviors that are shared because of the women's shared society. They all share the belief that women must have children to be full women in the society and that having many children is a blessing. This opinion was tempered in the younger women, however, who also focused on the convenience of smaller families. One such younger woman, Paz, said, "I also got an operation. Children are a lot of work. After my boy [was born] my husband said it would be best if I got an operation so I would have no more. . . . They are tiring. Children are a lot of work."

These women's reproductive habitus includes practices of prenatal care for mothers-to-be—traditional birth or obstetric care—as well as the behaviors surrounding the birth itself: the techniques of birth and obstetrics (Mauss 1973). The *sobada*—traditional massage—is a significant part of women's reproduction in this region. *Sobadas* are carried out during pregnancy by a tradition birth attendant who palpates the woman's abdomen. Genoveva, who moonlighted as a *sobadora* and *partera*, said, "As you feel how the baby is developing, well, we [slowly] turn it so that it comes [out] properly." As Cristina said, regarding her experiences during pregnancy, "[The *partera*] will supposedly position the baby properly. Indigenous women carry heavy things, like wood or water, and the baby [can] move to the side." During the birth itself, the *sobada* can help ease a woman's contractions and relax her for an easier birth experience. It is also important in the postpartum, both to help the woman return to normal and to ease an infant's colic.

Mauss's techniques of the body also include birthing positions; he especially confronts the idea of normalcy, and how birthing in one position—on one's knees among the women in Amatlán, for instance—is "no more normal than doing so in other positions" (79) such as in the supine position in Western obstetrics. Indeed, most of the traditional birth attendants were uncomfortable by the biomedical position as they felt it exposed the woman too much to public view, by showing "everything to everyone," as Refugio noted. Many women compare the different birth options available, judging each one as modern or primitive. As Adelina, an older woman in her sixties, said disparagingly, "They used to be born like little pigs, because they were born on the ground."

The reproductive habitus produces different types of people and interactions between members of a society. For instance, Mauss writes about the postpartum period and the rearing of children, going into detail about mother-child contact through carrying and nursing. He states that children carried for their first few years of infancy and who experience extended breastfeeding have "contact with [their] mother quite unlike [our] children's" (79). A habitus such as this would produce not only different relations between members of the group, but also, possibly, different types of people, for whom physical contact or emotional closeness brings pleasure.

The mothers I interacted with in Amatlán are some of the most loving and nurturing I have seen: they carry their infants constantly, rarely setting them down even for sleep; they are indulgent but do not spoil their children; they rarely use physical punishment; instead they instill reason and sensibility in their children; and they use good humor and gentle joking to overcome difficult behavior. In all the years I have lived with these women, I rarely saw an out-of-control child or one who had tantrums—instead I saw children who from early ages learned responsibility and limits. Children learn the practices of village life—carrying water, fetching firewood, lighting the fire to cook, making *masa* and tortillas, using a machete, tending the animals—through socialization at their mothers' knees. All the young children I met during my years of fieldwork stayed close to their mother's world and learned the intricacies of living in Amatlán. This was epitomized by the giving to Betina and Yanine—*Comadre* Alicia's youngest daughter and her granddaughter (Estela's daughter), who were eight and two years old respectively—the duty of going to the stream to fetch water. Because both girls knew to be careful and responsible by the water, there was no fear of an accident or drowning. Such behaviors are the embodiment of the women's mothering and reproductive habitus.

The institutions that the women interact with—social, political, economic, and medical—expect certain behaviors from the women's reproduction. Many of these behaviors are contradictory, and they are embodied in the women's daily lives. The women are at once assertive but obedient, informed but docile, sexually liberated but sporadic users of contraception. And in these expectations of behaviors, the habitus of "rational, self-regulating 'hygienic citizenship'" is imposed on them (Mitchell 2006:352). All these expectations are meant to be embodied in the women until they become second nature. Similarly to the children Lisa Mitchell (2006) worked with in the Philippines, the women's "body and its composition, functions, and care have been tied to nation-building and citizenship" (352).

But the women of Amatlán do not simply absorb these expectations like sponges; instead they grapple with them and play with them (Bonfil Batalla 1996). The women adopt the necessary changes or the ones they see as attractive; they modify them and do not accept them monolithically. They absorb the practices that are useful to them, they accept the Oportunidades money eagerly, and they use humor to respond to difficulties in their interactions with institutional forces. The women's techniques "consist of an adaptation of the body to their use" (Mauss 1973:86), where stoicism and composure help them to navigate the difficulties they encounter in their interactions with physicians and other representatives of Mexican institutions. Within their niche, the women experience their reproductive habitus as a continual interaction between their dispositions, constraints, and possibilities of reality. Their reproductive choices are not limitless; even though conceivably there are limitless options for action, the women would not think of these options, and in this way they do not exist as possibilities (Douglas 1986).

Of Sueros *and Other Fluids: Birthing the Modern Way*

Within the system created by the nexus of Oportunidades and clinicians, where a concern exists for the public health and reproductive lives of indigenous, rural, and poor communities, the process of birth thus becomes especially important. In such efforts at modernizing maternity and childbearing, the state can reach into women's maternity and dictate the behaviors and how birth should take place (see, for instance, Jolly 1998; Manderson 1998). The polemical nature of childbirth within the discourses of development becomes illustrated by Celeste's particularly poignant birth story. Celeste, a teenage single-mother-to-be, was very embarrassed to give birth in the exposed horizontal position at the clinic, and she kept on trying to get up to give birth vertically. Nurse Juliana told me the story later:

> Some women are embarrassed. There was once a girl who came with her parents about seven years ago, but she did not let us touch her or anything; she did not let us check to see how dilated she was. And her parents supported her instead of telling her to pay attention to us. Finally the girl jumped off the bed and she ran to that post [a post at the fence around the clinic] and she held onto it and squatted down and began to push. I told her that I would not attend to her out there, and that if she did not come in and labor inside the clinic then she would have to leave. And she did not want to come in. . . . She left and had her child along the way.

She then stated that Celeste had also been very troublesome to the traditional birth attendant who had tried to help her with subsequent births. Concluding her story, she said,

> But, that girl was very irresponsible in that regard. She said she would have no more children and now she has about five. . . . Later on she did give birth here [at the clinic] normally, lying down, and without a *partera*. Maybe the first day [she behaved that way] because she did not know about the contractions. But her mother and father spoiled

her a lot; they spoiled her a lot, that is why she would do what she wanted. But outside [of this clinic] she [can't give birth] because if not who would be responsible for the outcome?

Because of the clinical boundaries, medical and Hippocratic responsibility ended at the clinic entrance, and so anything happening beyond (and in direct opposition to the medical orders) was the patient's own responsibility. So Celeste was irresponsible as a patient and mother: she disobeyed medical orders and thus her birth occurred at her own risk. In the nurse's view, it was illogical for Celeste to want to give birth outside of the "proper," "modern," and "normal" medical setting; such disregard for "correctness" is not allowed, and thus the disobedient person has to either comply with or be removed from the medical establishment. Juliana saw Celeste's noncompliance as a hindrance to development and, in effect, an attack against Juliana's efforts to help her.

Traditional birth attendants have historically been integral to the reproductive process in marginalized areas across the world. Lenore Manderson (1998), in her analysis of maternity in colonial Malaya, discusses how midwives acted as gatekeepers to biomedicine, determining the community's acceptance and compliance. Cosminsky's (2001) work in Guatemala sharply illustrates traditional birth attendants' importance within the various types of healers in Mesoamerica. Fraser (1995) shows how the African American midwife in the southern United States was all but eradicated at the beginning of the twentieth century. These midwives' practice was equated with other social ills. She refers to the process of substitution of black midwives by white clinicians as the "cultural hygienization of reproductive health care" (Fraser 1995:45).

Across Mexico, traditional birth attendants participate with women, through prenatal massages, throughout the labor and birth process, to the postpartum period (Huber and Sandstrom 2001), which in Amatlán has included a cleansing bath for the mother and newborn (Sandstrom 1991; Smith-Oka 2008). The forms of birth women experience ultimately shape their perceptions of maternity and modernity. A tussle exists between tradition and the past, represented by the *parteras* (traditional birth attendants), and modernity and the future, represented by the clinicians. Receiving biomedical reproductive care is viewed as a necessary step toward achieving development and modernity. For the women of Fraser's (1995) study, to receive biomedical care was seen as a transition to having modern bodies and modern minds—even if such modernity came at the expense of traditional forms of knowledge. As research among anthropologists of reproduction has shown (Craven 2005; MacDonald 2006; Dudgeon 2012; Maraesa 2012; Smith-Oka 2012), within the scope of problematic reproduction lie traditional birth attendants and the women who go to them. Biomedical institutions would argue that engagement in traditional birth is not only "unmodern" but also extremely risky—additional "transgressions" against responsibility and motherhood.

A skilled birth attendant (SBA) is defined by the World Health Organization (WHO) as "an accredited health professional—such as a midwife, doctor, or nurse—who has been educated and trained to proficiency in the skills needed to manage normal (uncomplicated) pregnancies, childbirth and the immediate postnatal period, and in the identification, management and referral of complications in women and newborns" (WHO 2008:1). Because traditional birth attendants (TBA) are not formally trained, they are not considered skilled. The term "midwife," while often used as a catchall term for any nonphysician who attends births, actually refers to a trained professional.[9]

I find this terminological distinction used by larger health and development bodies especially interesting. This is a distinction that boils down to a binary between skilled and traditional, modern and outdated. Brigitte Jordan's (1993:196) term "cosmopolitan obstetrics" is particularly apt, especially in contrast to "ethno-obstetrics"—the former embodying authoritative and legitimate knowledge and the latter one neither. Stacy Leigh Pigg (1997) shows how the classification and naming of local health practitioners by development projects devalues local knowledge while placing development ideas at the locus of modern and authoritative forms of knowledge. Words, she maintains, "organize actions" (1997:233). And while in Mexico the term *partera* remains in use, concern among the medical personnel about traditional birth attendant–assisted births is very prevalent. As Juliana, the nurse, stated, "It's just that if they are not trained they do not know." Thus attendance by these practitioners is discouraged because, who wants traditional citizens in a Third World nation?

Long before the Millennium Development Goals were created, Mexico aimed to absorb, reeducate, or dissolve the *parteras* practicing in villages and urban places across the country. To achieve this absorption effort, Mexico embarked on removing traditional birth attendants from practice in the early twentieth century, often denigrating them as vestiges of a superstitious and unhygienic past (Stern 1999). As Cosminsky (2001) points out in her review of birth attendants in Mexico and Guatemala, within the medicalization process, the role of TBAs is increasingly secularized, slowly losing its ritual or religious aspects.

Through the certification of midwives, the Mexican government's intention has been to bring modernization and medical health care to the remote corners of the country. It was not until the 1970s, however, that the government began to recognize midwives' potential to reproductive health care. Certified traditional birth attendants were frequently betwixt and between both systems of health and could become the local implementers of the long arm of the government. Paola Sesia (1996), in her work among indigenous *parteras* in the Mexican state of Oaxaca, shows how traditional birth attendance was restructured to "incorporate" it into the national health system, but only those practices that would pose no threat, ultimately decontextualizing them from the larger cultural logic (Freyermuth and Sesia 2006). This system captured and brought midwifery practices into the national health system by modifying them and making them acceptable to biomedicine. But, as Jenkins (2003) points out, this bridging practice is simply a stopgap measure until all women can be covered by biomedical health care. The ultimate purpose is not to incorporate alternative forms of birth attendance into a society, but rather to keep them only until "better" options are available. Pigg (1997) demonstrates how development systems frequently use this process as a means to dismantle different cultural realities in the same breath as they "learn" about them and take them into account. This is perhaps not that different from the process of *indigenismo*.

The certification courses for *parteras* have usually been aimed at improving their skills in prenatal care and getting them to incorporate greater hygiene during the birth and immediate postpartum period, and especially at enabling them to identify high-risk and crisis situations. Brigitte Jordan (1993:170) uses the term "upgrade" to refer to the process of changing the practitioners' knowledge and having them "learn" about correct forms of perinatal care. She describes the mind-numbing courses that TBAs receive during the process of certification, where much of the emphasis is on lecture-style learning of reproductive processes and definitions. In the three decades since Jordan's observations, not much has changed in these courses, except for the inclusion of a practical "hands-on" element where *parteras* can witness "how birth is done" in a clinical setting. Refugio was particularly critical of the birth position used at hospital settings, stating, "The doctor in Xalapa told us . . . that it should be born like this [opens her arms wide to indicate open legs in stirrups]. But then they showed us all [the parts] of that poor woman. We would all stand in front of her and we would see the baby being born. That is very embarrassing." She expressed this extreme discomfort on many occasions, shuddering at the shame and comparing the medical position unfavorably to the kneeling position she used, which gave women much more dignity and kept them from being exposed "for all the world to see."

Professionalization courses usually give birth attendants a certificate of their training as well as a medical kit filled with "tools of the trade" (Jordan 1993:180), such as gloves, gauze, measuring tape, thermometer, a scale to weigh the baby, a Pinard stethoscope to hear the fetal heart rate, vitamin K for the baby's eyes, and soap, among other things. For Lourdes, being certified not only gave her the tools for her practice, but also the external validation from medical professionals meant that she could consider herself a better birth attendant. She said, "In Poza Rica they treated us like doctors because what the [doctors] can't do, we can. . . . That is why they told us that it is good that we work and do what they can't do." She stated that she was registered in Poza Rica as a *partera*, yet she added sadly,

> But there are very few births here nowadays; they go to Tepatepec to give birth, to the clinic there or if not they go to get operated at [the hospital in] Chicón, to have a cesarean to have no more children. I work daily. There in Poza Rica they gave me things to help when [a woman] gives birth. . . . Many [women] come to me! It's just that they know that I can, that's why they come. . . . They come to me from very far away; they know me. But many now go to the clinic, they no longer want [birth] at home. But it is better at home. When they gave us the course in Poza Rica they told us that it is better at home.

It was not quite so evident, however, that the local clinicians agreed with Lourdes's idea that birth was better at home. The scope of practice allowed to certified *parteras* seems to vary across regions and even within medical centers, as some centers very strictly divide between medicine and *parteras*, while others allow TBAs to attend births within the clinical setting (for example, Doctora Felipa often allowed *parteras* to attend to their patients within the clinic itself, while the hospital in Llano would not allow a *partera* to accompany her patient into the emergency room).

While certification can bring legitimacy, often the attendants' authoritative knowledge is contested or dismissed by clinicians, ultimately making TBAs subordinate to biomedicine (Cosminsky 2001). Most of the local clinicians, while sometimes admiring the abilities of the birth attendants, frequently expressed concern about their knowledge and techniques. Nurse Juliana at Tepatepec said about traditional birth attendants in general, "They are very good; they can really detect multiple pregnancies, twinning, the [baby's] position, and they are good at attending the birth." Despite this admiration, she did express many reservations about their abilities, especially if they were not certified. She stated,

> There are many dangers [that can kill the baby]. I have often seen the [*parteras*] so preoccupied with the expulsion of the placenta that they only later clean the baby. And it should not be like that. Those are the risks. . . . Sometimes they bring their patients here if they can't help them. And it is important for them to see how a birth is managed in the clinic. . . . Yes, for a *partera* my concern would be hygiene. There is no ideal space for birth [at their home]. And a birth requires lots of hygiene to prevent infections. Also, if a baby is coming out wrong [for example with a] lack of oxygen, the *partera* doesn't know how to act at that moment and there can be a death, both maternal and of the baby.

Doctora Felipa at the Ixhuatlán clinic seemed particularly concerned about the risk involved in TBA births:

> There is always risk, and then onto that we add the fact that the [birth place's] conditions are not the best, or if the *partera* uses medicines that she is not trained to use. In those cases the only thing that has worth is the experience they have to manipulate [the vaginal opening] because, wow, I have nothing but admiration for them, they do not allow it to tear. But it is their experience that has allowed them to do that. But from that to them having actual knowledge, that they don't.

Felipa's words are particularly interesting. She admires many of the manipulative techniques used by the TBAs as well as their knowledge of local ideas, yet she does not give their knowledge equal status to her own. She dismisses "the relevance of any other mode of being in the world" (Jordan 1993:184). Claire Wendland, in her dual work as an obstetrician and medical anthropologist, stated that physicians believe that they have "knowledge," while their patients have "culture" (personal communication, November 17, 2011). This binary nature explains much of these interactions between the clinicians and their patients, so that even when traditional birth attendants do become certified they are still considered to be untrained and with less knowledge than is safe for their practice. It once again juxtaposes notions of tradition versus modernity and gives primacy to what Jordan refers to as cosmo*political* obstetrics, where a particular distribution of power is enforced across social and cultural divisions (Jordan 1993:196).

For the women and clinicians in this region, part of being a modern mother is to have had a modern birth. Such a birth would be clinically based, with the woman lying on a gurney in an operating room and her legs in stirrups; there would also be the use of Pitocin, intravenous fluids, and technology (such as heart monitor). Within this schema then, traditional birth attendants fall outside of development. Not only are they unmodern, they are also risky. And how can a risky, unmodern birthing situation lead to the production of modern and fully functioning citizens?

The conflict between development and tradition was not solely in the realm of the medical profession. The women themselves also felt the tussle between their roots and their interest in modern medical care. Altagracia perhaps described the local concern with birth attendants the most vividly:

> And like that there is a great pain, I remember. And you have to call for the [*partera*] to come to look after you. Here inside [the house]. Not even a rag will you put down. Like that we would give birth, like animals. Like that the [baby's] head would fall [onto] the mud, and [the] blood. Nowadays they give birth in the hospital [and] they bathe them right away. . . . Like that we would give birth. We would just call the *partera*. We never went with the doctor. Like that we would give birth, like animals. We had lots of children.

All of Altagracia's eight children were born at home with a *partera*. She is in her late fifties and is one of the few remaining women who still wear the traditional skirt and embroidered blouse. As a Pentecostal she was often critical of any type of health care that was not prayer based. While she received medical care from the clinic and had even had surgery a few years previously, she preferred to care for her illnesses at home, using prayer and simple home remedies and medicinal plants.

Most of women's concern with TBAs was the fact that they did not use *suero*—intravenous fluids—which for people in Mexico is often akin to the most modern medical care, practically a magic elixir—and the fact that they relied on the kneeling position for birth. Frida said, "[At the clinic] they give you *suero* and you'll see that it will not hurt when you give birth. Here with the *partera* it does hurt because she does not give you *suero*. . . . And with the *suero* you give birth faster. Like that it is better with the doctor." This sentiment was echoed by other women, particularly those who were in their early to late thirties, who had the experience of giving birth with a TBA for their eldest children and at the clinic with their youngest. Paz was especially critical of the ways that *parteras* managed birth. She said,

> [My daughter] was born in Ixhuatlán, because here it is with a *partera* and, well, they have to cut you down there so you can give birth properly, and the *partera* does not do that. . . . But here with a *partera* you are not allowed to rest. She just tells you to push and push and it is very tiring. At the clinic [that does] not [happen]. There you have pain but they give you *suero*. . . . Yes, the doctor gives you an injection so that it comes out faster. He puts it into the *suero*. . . . And you get some pain, but the baby comes out soon. They say that with the *partera* it takes longer. The baby does not come out right away.

The traditional position for giving birth in this area is by kneeling on the ground, often having the support of the husband's arms or a rope tied to the rafters from which a woman can hold on and bear down. Refugio described her practice proudly, stating,

> They kneel and they hold on like this [points to the wooden side of the shed next to the kitchen] and the man holds her like this [indicates that he is behind the woman and holds her by the torso, below her breasts] and well, they stand above a plastic sheet. And if necessary I ask her if I can see if the kid is coming fine. And only I see this . . . not like the doctors. . . . If not they push and push and the kid does not come out. And the [doctors] don't use oil [to ease the passage]. With me, well, I catch the kid when it falls and I tie the cord and I cut it. And when they push again and the [placenta] comes then I also [bury it].

While gravity allows this sort of position to be very effective, opening up the woman's hips to allow the baby through, it can also be much more tiring for the woman, hurting her knees, arms, or waist. Ofelia, one of my *comadres*, who is a large woman with four children, was not particularly supportive of traditional birth attendance despite the fact that Lourdes is her mother-in-law.[10] She told me her birth stories one day in 2007 as we drank *refresco* (soft drinks) in her kitchen while she cooked a meal of her delicious, warm, and spicy *mole*. She said,

> I swelled up with Alana. It is better in the clinic. I swelled up because one does not know what to do during one's first pregnancy. I did not take vitamins. . . . I could not give birth normally with the *partera*. On swelling up, the part where the baby comes out closes up. I had to give birth with a private doctor. It was already nighttime. He cut me down there and he gave me some *suero*. It will give you strength so the baby is born. . . . With Andrés I was already fine. I tried to give birth here but I also couldn't. I was frightened. I gave birth in Llano [with a private doctor]. It was quick there. They also cut me. The three [children] were like that. . . . I prefer in clinics and hospitals. I am frightened at home with a *partera*. Because they do not let you rest. They are always telling you to push. Not [so with] the doctor; he [tells you to push] only when it hurts. . . . I think that [it is better] lying down. They open your legs and they have two iron rods to hold you. And kneeling hurts your knees; you get tired. There [at the clinic] you just push. Not here with the *partera*.

As Jenkins (2003) found with TBAs in Costa Rica, Mexican traditional birth attendants have been transformed by larger forces into relics of bygone times while simultaneously being reframed by changing local values and meanings about midwifery. The lack of respect felt from all parties has an effect on their self-value, ultimately affecting their practice. Lourdes draws on prayers to Santa Partera (Saint Midwife) to keep her from harm, while Refugio swallows her disappointment, stating, "I am not opposed to a woman who has complications going to the clinic.[11] I am not going to tell her to stay with me if I can't help her. But they used to come to me from very far away. Not anymore, since they go to the clinic. But it is better that way; I am tired."

Cristina, the mother of five children, expressed concerns that reflect many of the other villagers' notions of modernity and parteras. She had some of her first children with a TBA and her last daughter with medical attendance. She said,

> It is not recommended [to go] to a *partera*. In the past we knew nothing. If there is no money you stay at home. . . . My mother did not let me give birth with a *partera*. She said it is riskier. . . . With the *partera* you are curled up with your knees on the ground. With the doctor

you are lying down. It is more comfortable with a doctor than with a *partera*. It is always better with a doctor.

In these women's words can be found many themes revolving around development and modernity. Modernity for the women is about comfort, whether through having a painless birth as Frida mentioned, or from lying back during labor, as Cristina and Ofelia recalled. *Suero* becomes the all-important lifeline for modern birth and a very personal material object that can empower an anxious individual (Whyte et al. 2002). As with injections in Uganda, explored by Whyte et al. (2002), *suero* is an example of how medical technology is shaped by the particular cultural setting. Through the connection to the bottle of fluids, the women become increasingly modern. *Suero* stands for the "powerful substances and procedures of biomedicine" (Whyte et al. 2002:111), which marry the material, the social, and the symbolic "in a complex web of association," as Mauss would put it (Whyte et al. 2002:112). It is a very tangible way for the women to literally bring modernity into their bodies, emphasizing that it gives them strength and helps to make the birth faster and less painful.[12] In a sense, *suero* allows for the transformation, the metamorphosis, of the indigenous woman into developed woman through the entry of these fluids.

Development is also about being part of the market economy, as Cristina points out by saying that only if you have money will you go to the clinic. If you have no alternative then you will give birth at home. It is those with no money, the poorest, or the "animals" in Altagracia's comments, who are the most unmodern. While giving birth at the clinic is practically free, there is a tremendous cost in getting to the clinic, especially in the middle of the night, when the cost of transport increases exponentially. These women's concept of modernity varies significantly from what the physicians would term a modern birth, where the emphasis is on hygiene, control, technology, authority, or sterility—not comfort—or at least not the women's comfort. Indeed, these women's idea of comfort runs counter to the idea of comfort in the global North, where it is the element of choice and the luxury of a birth plan that provides the laboring woman the greatest comfort. For the women birthing in Ixhuatlán de Madero, a birth choice is rarely an option.

While we can observe that the women feel the tussle between their birth beliefs and wanting to be modern, there is also a sense of being pressured into going to the clinic. Even women who disdained traditionally attended birth, such as Cristina or Ofelia, stated that there was pressure from the clinic to give birth there. As Estela, one of my youngest and most recent *comadres*, who has two children under the age of five, said to me, "Here in the clinic they no longer want it to be done that [traditional] way. And so [for my son] I did not ask [a *partera*] and I went to the hospital in Llano. They don't like [children] to be born with a *partera*." This sentiment was echoed by Alicia, her mother, who put the issue into broader context, stating, "My three [oldest] children were born here in Amatlán, simply with a *partera*. . . . With Betina [her youngest] I went to the clinic. At that time they were already forcing us to go, because we already were receiving Oportunidades. And we have to check at the clinic." Even Juana, one of the most avid supporters of traditional birth attendance and plant-based home remedies in the village and whose eight children were all born at home, stated,

> Now there are few [women who give birth here]. Now they all go [to the clinic]. . . . Nowadays the doctor does not want them to give birth here; they should go there to give birth. It's just that there a baby is born and they inject them. They look after it. Now a baby no longer dies. Before they would die from *tentsocopale*.[13] Now as there is a doctor it is less work; they look after [the baby].

Juana's words encapsulate the state's central role in reproduction: the state takes the baby as soon as it is born, and it is injected with biomedical products that will keep it safe and make it modern. The physicians bring children into the light of the state.

Apparent from the women's words about the type of births they have had is a crux of the issue of motherhood and modernity. *Parteras* represent the past. Though they might still be sought for reproductive and sexual issues, they are less often called on to care for a woman's birth. They have been reconstructed in such a way that simply to be attended by a *partera* is to become old-fashioned or outdated. By going to a *partera* one becomes passé one's self. It is the modern mothers who go to physicians and clinics. Each of these birthplaces creates particular types of mothers. While there is no outright value judgment on good and bad mothers based on going to physicians or *parteras*, there is a strong connection between birth context and modernity, which becomes reflected in motherhood. As I have shown, if a woman, such as Dulce, becomes a mother through traditional birth-attended care she is considered old-fashioned and unmodern. A woman, such as Cristina, who becomes a mother through physician-centered care, is seen as forward looking and modern. Modern mothers are perceived to translate this modernity into success for themselves and their children—modern mothers speak Spanish, dress in nonindigenous manner, have fewer children, and understand the importance of education. Their children are seen as more likely to finish school and migrate for jobs or further education, thereafter sending money back to their family in the village.

Because of state policies such as Oportunidades that in effect demand that women (and their families) receive health care in medical settings, women have little choice but to accept that their reproductive care will come from biomedicine, or if they resist, and give birth with *parteras*, the state sees them as making bad choices that will affect both them and their children. They are perceived as noncompliant. Women who do this are seen as bad mothers, and they are blamed for their choices. Beatriz, a nurse at the hospital in Llano de Enmedio, said to me, "But [women] don't reflect upon the risk that each pregnancy carries. . . . They do not measure the consequences [going to a *partera*] can bring." These words illustrate the opposing ideas regarding traditional birth attendance. Women who have physician-attended births do so out of a desire to comply with clinic orders and to aim for modernity. Risk and its analysis are not part of their preference set. Their decision making is complex and does take several factors into account—such as comfort, modernity, safety, and risk. Yet for the clinicians, any decision that does not conform to their view is a reason to point to these women and affirm their own beliefs about the intractable nature of the indigenous peasantry.

In my earlier description of Celeste's birth, one can see how the ways the objectives of Oportunidades are carried out by the clinicians are often in direct opposition to local birthing practices. This is moreover the case because the medicalization of birthing in Mexico in health centers uses the model of women birthing horizontally. And while there are movements in Mexico to change this practice and ensure that women have options for birth position, these movements have not affected policy. There is no logical reason why women should not be able to give birth vertically in a health center; traditional and modern medicine should not be mutually exclusive categories—as indeed they are not at several hospitals across the country—for instance, the hospital in the town of Cuetzalan in Puebla[14]—where traditional healers and birth attendants work in the same hospital as biomedical personnel.

"There are no more children": Stratified Reproduction

Indigenous, marginalized, and low-income women in Mexico exist within a system of stratified reproduction, where their reproductive futures are valued only if they produce the acceptable low number of children and if they are "good mothers" to those children. The evaluation of women's motherhood is defined by the national Mexican perspective. This evaluation particularly focuses on women's fulfillment of "traditional" social roles and responsibilities and emphasizes normatively ascribed maternal responsibilities. The only form of motherhood encouraged by the state is one that sees the truth in the Mexican ideal of the right number of children and who has eschewed her "ignorant," indigenous ways. Through a combination of biopower—insidious forms of self-surveillance and self-discipline—and overt or dominant power emanating from the state, these women refashion their bodily practices and match their desires to those of the mainstream.

Whiteford and Manderson (2000) point out that policies aimed at maternal and child health, for instance, have always operated based on socioeconomic class. As in Mexico's puericulture and Oportunidades, middle-class and imperial values predominate in these programs; they achieve their expansion through surveillance of people's behaviors through home visits and by inspectors, medical staff, and welfare workers, who also convey the desired values to the populations lacking them.

Oportunidades creates desires in their enrolled populations, which explains how people's bodies and actions are manipulated and managed, resulting in their docility. A docile body is easy to control, easy to bend to one's will. And despite the purported intentions of Oportunidades to give more choice and freedom to women, it has become part of this system of structural violence whose primary aim is "no longer to protect the freedom of each individual [. . .] but rather to assume responsibility for the very manner in which the individual manages his life" (Ewald 1986:8). The women have internalized the self-regulation and have formed themselves into subjects. Frida, who embodies the struggles many of the women face by being simultaneously strong willed and powerless, bluntly said, "I would prefer to receive no money than [continue] to be asked to do so much [in order to receive it]."

Kate Goldade (2007) provides a fascinating example of the creation of citizenship and docile bodies in her work among Nicaraguan immigrants in Costa Rica. She explores how migrant reproduction has become a focus for processes of defining Costa Rican citizenship and limiting or accessing related entitlements. Using in-depth ethnographic narratives, she shows how undocumented migrant Nicaraguan women parlay reproductive strategies to achieve cultural citizenship. Goldade's work is a perfect illustration of stratified reproduction, a term used by Shellee Colen (1995) to describe the ways that certain populations are encouraged and empowered to reproduce while others are characterized as reproductive threats to society and thus disempowered to reproduce. Ginsburg and Rapp (1995:3) starkly point out that stratified reproduction "helps us to see the arrangements by which some reproductive futures are valued while others are despised." Leo Chavez (2004) confronts the discourse of stratified reproduction among Latinas in the United States and shows how equating certain groups with dangerous, pathological, and abnormal reproductive behaviors has very real political and economic consequences.

Cecilia Van Hollen (2003:166) uses the wonderful phrase "maneuvering development" to refer to first, "how development apparatuses maneuver individuals and groups to adopt new sets of ideas and practices in an attempt to fashion modern subjects," and second, how the people who are the targets of these programs maneuver "within and around these discourses in ways which collude with, resist, or alter the discourses." It is in the clinical encounters between the women of Amatlán and the medical staff that one can see the women's development being maneuvered by the development apparatus to fashion modern subjects; these groups have been classified as "less developed" and thus, as Van Hollen (2003:167) puts it, their minds must be reformed and, most particularly, their bodily practices must be transformed. In Van Hollen's research in India, it is low-income women who are the targets of development projects implemented by physicians who frequently condemn their maternal health practices. In that example, the women are also a captive audience for development, though the timeframe is shorter than for the women of Amatlán as it tends to be confined to the postpartum period of hospital recovery, as opposed to several years of receiving cash transfers from the government.

Many of the implementers of development projects interested in changing women's roles and behaviors have a strong faith in the development narrative of progress yet often feel discouraged about being able to achieve actual change, feeling that it is an uphill battle to "convince 'these women' to change their ways" (Van Hollen 2003:172). "We tell them, but they don't listen" is a frequent lament of the clinicians in Amatlán. To convince women to comply, clinicians will often lay out their faults in public. For instance, at one of the information sessions at the clinic, "the nurse congratulated all the women [at the meeting] because almost all of them had had the operation and were going to have no more children. But [then] she pointed to one woman and told her that she had too many children and that she should have the operation." Such public singling out serves not only to embarrass the woman into compliance but also serves as a warning to other women that disobedience carries consequences. Her good citizenship—and being "like us," as Goldade (2007) states—is assured through her obedience. Such treatment is not unusual in medical centers for low-income populations, as Maternowska (2006:78) discovered in her research at a clinic of a slum in Haiti. She points out that such curt, and almost rude, behavior toward patients "conforms to the society's dominant expectations about appropriate behavior towards the poor."

So how exactly is the Amatlán women's maternity a problem? For all intents and purposes, the women are quite compliant: they are all enrolled in Oportunidades and thus are slowly being "resocialized" to have fewer children; they tend to participate readily in the clinic activities—albeit with the sword of Damocles hanging over their heads; and they participate as *ciudadanas*—citizens—in the maintenance of the visible cleanliness and order of the village. In small ways, the women can be seen as problematic, for not attending prenatal care regularly, for instance, or not participating in *pláticas* when asked to, or not feeding their children correctly. In the eyes of authority, these behaviors are only small parts of a larger problem. The larger problem is the women's ability to reproduce and their indigenousness.

These two factors—being female and indigenous—compounded by the women's poverty—immediately classify them as problematic for the advancement of Mexican society. Because to be poor, indigenous, and female means that one is a person who rapidly reproduces and thus produces many more mouths to feed. Such mouths to feed then become the problem of the larger state. Regardless of how many children an indigenous woman actually wants or has, simply by being indigenous she is classified as a dangerous reproducer who must be stopped for the benefit of society. This mindset is pervasive throughout Mexico, and, indeed, in many parts of the global South, which shows that it is the poor population who the government believes are the problem. It frowns on their reproduction.

Only the people at the bottom of the social hierarchy carry the stigma of being problematic. In the paternalistic system in which they exist, not only is their reproduction feared, but it must also be controlled. Though family planning and contraception options are provided to low-income populations at government clinics ostensibly to provide reproductive choice, underlying this policy is the larger guiding principle of controlling problematic reproducers. It is within these policies of stratified reproduction that much more aggressive practices and programs arise, such as the *Programa de Anticoncepción Posevento Obstétrico*, the Post-Obstetric Event Contraceptive Program (Castro 2004). This program was implemented in the late 1990s to encourage low-income women to receive a tubal ligation immediately after birth. The logic was that the woman was already at the hospital and thus would be saved the inconvenience of coming back later to be sterilized. This approach also guaranteed that the women would not vanish from medical sight and control. This is a very effective way to obtain compliance and eventual obedience, as the woman is a "captive" audience (as Van Hollen observed among women in India), and her reproductive life can effectively be brought to a close.

States always seek to shape reproduction, especially women's bodies, sexuality, and maternity. Women's biological ability to reproduce is thus seen as the embodiment of disobedience, because short of forced sterilization, the state cannot reach into the bedroom in the way it wants. Oportunidades at the locus of the clinic ingeniously circumvents this dilemma and can have a hand in managing and shaping the sexual and reproductive lives of its beneficiary women.

CHAPTER 3

Conflicted Relationships at Home and at the Clinic

A POSTER HANGS PROMINENTLY IN THE CLINIC AT TEPATEPEC. A PICTURE of a happy extended indigenous family—mother, father (carrying their one daughter), and grandparents—reads "*¡Que no te discriminen! Tienes derecho a que te traten con respeto. Si alguien te trata mal, o te condiciona la prestación de un servicio, repórtalo a Oportunidades*" (No one should discriminate against you! You have the right to be treated with respect. If anyone treats you badly, or places conditions on [your receiving] services, report it to Oportunidades). It then lists various toll-free numbers that can be dialed. Perhaps this poster shows that the government is becoming aware of the drawbacks of conditional cash. It might also reflect the class and social structure of Mexico, where social programs have been historically used by the elite classes to control the behaviors (and votes) of low-income populations. Embedded within the structure of Oportunidades is that women must be obedient to the program, to clinicians, and to husbands, or face consequences. This reality is deeply ironic as it runs counter to the apparent goals of empowering the women by making them beneficiaries of the cash transfers.

There is a direct impact on the women's reproductive health that emerges as a result of the conditions of Oportunidades, whose ground evaluators have their own professional missions and goals. For the clinicians at the clinics and hospitals, population control and demographics are key objectives—for both medical and pedagogical ends. It is at the clinic where all these unintended consequences and the confluence of all these state-level forces—Oportunidades, population control, health-service provision—are enacted on women's bodies, demanding compliance.

Oportunidades is very clear about the rights of its enrolled families. Among the many rights that the families have—including access to basic health services and educational facilities—there is also the explicit right to reproductive freedom. Beneficiary families are, theoretically, permitted to have as few or as many children as they wish—as stated in the Mexican Constitution.[1] This right is included on posters and other informative material provided to the enrolled families. These state very clearly that women can choose to have as many children as they want because they have reproductive freedom. Though there is no actual connection between Oportunidades and CONAPO—the National Population Council—the intermediary ministries of health (SSA, IMSS, and so on) are the ones that implement population and family-planning policies. In this way, the idea of full reproductive freedom espoused by Oportunidades is cleverly circumvented, and thus the population policies become intimately connected and implemented among the enrolled mothers, who are also the poorest members of society.

The Population Policy Mission

After establishing the General Population Law in 1936, Mexico experienced a demographic momentum (Cabrera 1994) whereby the "right" type of Mexicans were encouraged to marry and to increase their birthrate. Schoolbooks included ideologies of Mexico's greatness and its large population. Monetary rewards were given to families with many children, which also gained them social recognition. The sale of contraceptives was prohibited. And some states even established a tax on unmarried people over twenty-five years old and on divorced or widowed people without children (Cabrera 1994).

Because of the pronatalist push, Mexico's population increased exponentially from the early twentieth to the early twenty-first century (Braff 2008). Over these one hundred years, the population grew from 13.6 million people to over 103 million, a sevenfold growth. From 1900 to 1974, the country experienced an annual growth rate of 1.1 percent and an emphasis on urbanization. From 1974 to 2000, concern arose about the large population (in 1970, Mexico had fifty million people) and its associated problems and dangers. From 1974 to 2000, the population growth rate was almost 3.5 percent. By 2000, the country had a growth rate of 1.4 percent annually, which was almost the same as the growth rate for the beginning of the twentieth century (Ordorica Mellado 2006).

During Gustavo Díaz Ordaz's presidency from 1964 to 1970, in a directly anti-Malthusian frame, the rapid population growth was hailed as the vehicle for Mexico's move into a modern and developed nation. However, Díaz Ordaz's successor, Luis Echeverría, began to notice the cracks emerging with unchecked population growth. These cracks showed how overpopulation could "clash with the social goals of the revolution" (Laveaga 2007:22). Echeverría's response was to implement frenetic anti-growth population policies across the country, most notable of which was the establishment of the Consejo Nacional de Población (CONAPO; National Population Council). It stated that its main role was to improve maternal and infant health standards while implementing "correct forms of family planning" among the "growing number of peasants" (Laveaga 2007:21).

Because of these population policies, fecundity rates have dropped markedly. The National Population Council estimates that the population growth will gradually taper off, with the country reaching a negative population growth by the year 2050 (CONAPO 2012). These projections are based on the increasing percentage of women of reproductive age who are practicing contraception, which increased from 70.7 percent to 73.2 percent between 2000 and 2004 (CONAPO 2004). CONAPO projects an even greater increase in contraception over the next few years. The council's data shows that the greatest levels of poverty and marginalization in Mexico are in areas with high death rates and young marriage ages, where women become pregnant with their first child while very young, and where there is a low use of family planning and contraceptive methods. Additionally, the regions and social groups of Mexico that register the highest development rates and standards of living are in the highest stages of demographic transition and experience lower death rates, women marrying and giving birth at an older age, and a higher use of family-planning methods (CONAPO 2004:5).

Childbearing is a legal right in Mexico, which is coupled with the right to receive family planning. The Mexican government uses the official discourse of family planning to promote women's rights, as per the 1994 International Conference on Population and Development (ICPD) in Cairo. In recent years, this mission has been accompanied by an increase of family-planning programs among the most marginalized populations in Mexico (urban and poor). This is viewed as a strategy to fight poverty (Nazar Beutelspacher et al. 2003:218).

These policies show the concern that the Mexican government has regarding population growth. Even though fecundity rates have significantly dropped, the government continues to be fearful of high population. These fears are not directed at the general population but rather at the populations that are more economically vulnerable, that is, poor, rural, and indigenous populations, and those lacking formal education. Admittedly, this is partly because on the whole, groups of higher socioeconomic status have smaller families. According to Tuirán et al. (2002), the groups of lower socioeconomic status are far behind other groups in the demographic transition in Mexico; they also have the highest levels of unsatisfied demand of contraceptive products. The population policy of the country aims to reduce this situation with short and long term strategies; they aim to do this by increasing access to contraceptives and by "articulating their operation with the broadest strategies for social and human development and for overcoming poverty" (Tuirán et al. 2002:33).

The Mexican government's fears are manifested in population policies that demonstrate the deepest notions of power. The "overly fertile" people's perceived noncompliance is rapidly ascribed to culturalist explanations of the ignorance and obstinacy of poor, indigenous people. For this reason, the state perceives itself as the only entity that can control these women's obstinate reproduction. The belief holds that if these women are too ignorant to know what is best for them, then the state needs to do it for them (Farmer 2006; Maternowska 2006).

Braff (2009) demonstrates in her work on fertility clinics in Mexico City that these perceptions about the reproduction of low-income populations exist across the country. Such perceptions shape the interaction between the physicians, the nurses, and the women who come to the clinics and hospitals in Ixhuatlán. The clinicians enthusiastically implement the national family-planning policy.[2] This information is usually imparted to reproductive-age women every time they attend the clinic. The medical opinion is that in order to protect the women from their high fertility (and to protect the country from the mouths of poor people), they have to be encouraged to contracept or to be sterilized so that they can lead richer and more fulfilling lives, by enjoying their newfound sexuality without the consequence of children. The number of children born into poverty can also be reduced. The concept of sexual freedom is a middle-class concept, however, and not necessarily applicable to marginalized women. It is most likely the fear of poverty that drives this belief and its associated policies.

Many of these population policies retain a core of neo-Malthusian orthodoxy, however. This orthodoxy equates high population growth with a depletion of resources; the purported solution has been to increase population control programs. Petchesky (1995) confronts this idea by stating that the ICPD discarded the neo-Malthusian language that framed population growth as the main cause of the economic and environmental crises. Instead, the language emphasized reproductive freedoms and rights. Petchesky states that the emphasis is now on the complexity of factors that lead to poverty, including women's low status, social and economic inequality, and the problematic patterns of distribution and consumption. It is thus not obvious that population, development, and social inequality fit together as Malthusian arguments assume they do.

"They forcibly sent her to be operated": *The Politics of Reproduction*

Only a few weeks into my first field season in Amatlán, I was faced with the concerns the women of the village had regarding their reproductive bodies. Esperanza and I were conversing about issues of health, and she reported that Lourdes had accompanied one of her female patients to Chicontepec[3], three hours away by car, where her patient was to give birth. I asked why the woman was taken to the hospital in Chicontepec instead of simply giving birth at home or in the clinic in Tepatepec, a fifteen-minute drive away. Esperanza put down the embroidery she was working on, gave me a quick glance, and answered:

> She has been taken there so that she can be sterilized, because the doctor [at the clinic in Tepatepec] told her to be operated so that she has no more children because she already has four. He has already prepared the papers for her to be taken. They forcibly sent her to be operated, because she has too many children. The doctor says [women] should only have two children.

This was the first of many references to force, sterilization, and coercion made by the women. What was evident was that the women saw this coercion located at the clinic and emerging from their interactions with physicians and nurses. As Blanca said, "Yes, people say that they forcibly operate. In the clinic they force you a lot. They always tell my mother to get an operation. She was [using] injections but then did not want to [continue], and then she had a little [boy]."

While there has been little reference in Mexico to the sorts of forced sterilization campaigns exhibited by other countries (for example in India and Peru), these women's concerns were indicative of a problem that was hiding in the shadows. What was perhaps most disquieting was that these women seemed troubled by, yet resigned, to this treatment. Over time it became apparent that this story was not unique but rather was part of all the women's experiences. Every woman I spoke with had some story to share about her feelings of being coerced or forced at some point in their reproductive lives. Alicia stated, "The [staff] at the clinic tell us over and over not to have more children. That then one cannot buy things for one's children and there is no money. They tried to convince me three times to have an operation. But I didn't want to. But they forcibly send others to . . . be operated. . . . That is why there aren't any children here." The women expressed, through their words and resignation, their very obvious concern with what they saw as stratified reproduction—where their reproduction and motherhood was denied or curtailed, while those of other groups was encouraged. As far as they were concerned, the physicians and nurses were directly responsible for curtailing their reproduction.

One way to understand the politics of reproduction is to address the interactions between the women and the clinicians at clinics and hospitals in the region. Delving into the training that Mexican nurses and physicians receive, into the marked ethnic differences between them and their patients, and into the politics of health, one can see that there will inevitably be a hierarchy established between the groups. In this way, one can see how noncompliance is viewed in the medical setting and how the staff uses their status to implement programs and procedures in their target population. It is in this context that the actual compliance or noncompliance of the women exists: women who have more than three children are seen as overly fertile and marked as problematic, while those who follow the population policies and have fewer children are hailed as paragons of modernity.

Juliana, the nurse in Tepatepec, felt it was her mission to educate all the women about contraceptive and family-planning options. She frequently bemoaned the existence of families: "with nine or ten children, or the woman who at 45 or older is still having [children], . . . or the girls who at 13 or 14 get pregnant." For her, someone like Blanca's mother, who at forty-four had given birth to her seventh child, was precisely the population she agonized over. She extolled the benefits of sterilization, stating, "Sometimes they joke and say that they would like another one [and say] 'but I have been operated.' They feel good. As I tell them, once they have the surgery they can enjoy their sexuality." Acknowledging that other factors could contribute to the women's decisions, she added, "I tell them what is done in the women's surgery and the one for men. Now, *they* do get frightened. . . . The men don't want to [get a vasectomy] because of machismo."

Decision making is not simply based on an individual's desire for something but exists within a larger complex of factors—in the case of the women, these factors include their own desires for their family's size and their husband's wishes and concerns regarding family planning, as well as the national population policies and their co-optation by the clinicians. All these factors work together synergistically to form a system that the women have to negotiate in their reproductive lives. None of these factors exists independently of the others, particularly because of the women's enrollment in Oportunidades, which requires their involvement in larger processes (both medical and educational) outside of their community. In short, because the women have come to depend on the regular cash stipends as guaranteed supplementary income, they are unable to oppose the supervisory medical staff, specifically when the latter use the conditions to promote national family-planning policies.

In the larger politics of reproduction, women's bodies are a battleground, where policies created in elegant city offices are executed in a blanket fashion on populations that are invisible, except for their "development" potential. These policies inadvertently affect local populations because of unforeseeable issues at the local and regional levels created by the various actors involved. I would like to make it clear I am not coming at this issue from an essentialist or pronatalist viewpoint that eschews family-planning and contraception options for women. Nor do I mean to suggest that indigenous women have no agency; instead I show that despite local negotiations, indigenous women of Mexico still live within a system that implies that they cannot, or will not, control their own reproduction, and that thus the state (or another authority) needs to do it for them (Maternowska 2006). As Paul Farmer (2006:xiii) states, "It is important that those seeking to improve services to the poor understand how class works in a society traversed by such steep grades of inequality."

At the Clinics and Hospitals

There are a variety of clinics and hospitals in the municipality of Ixhuatlán de Madero, ranging from the tiny clinics dotted around the region, frequently staffed by only one physician and one nurse, to the state-run hospital, which has a staff of several dozen clinicians as well as operating rooms, delivery rooms, and other accouterments of a modern hospital. In addition to state-run clinics, there are several small *consultorios* (private practices) that charge higher fees to their patients. These physicians primarily attend the needs of the middle class; only in a great emergency do the poorer people go there, and even in these cases, they tend to be people with a little bit more money than the truly destitute.

Medical health care arrived in this region in the late 1970s; it consisted of a small, irregularly staffed *centro de salud* (government-run rural clinic) in Ixhuatlán. In the late 1990s, the government created an impetus to make medical care accessible to more rural areas and thus small *centros de salud* sprang up in accessible and well-connected areas. All the communities in this area are in the care of government-run clinics, though for many of these populations this means that people have to walk more than two hours to reach the clinic, sometimes having to ford streams and deep rivers to get there. These are arduous journeys that are undertaken only in the direst of situations. Women in labor have been carried for several hours to reach the clinic, sometimes dying before arrival; victims of snakebites have to hobble for many kilometers in the hope of reaching the physician in time; and the very old and very sick frequently lose hope because of the great distance. One woman stated, "One time a woman died in [this *partera's*] arms. She kept on telling her, 'you will give birth, you will give birth' and she didn't want to take her to the clinic. She didn't like to go there. And the woman was not giving birth and finally they took her to the clinic but she died on the way. That's why [that *partera*] sends [her patients] to the clinic if the birth is not [progressing]."

In some of these more remote villages are *casas de salud* (houses of health). These are small, simple structures built by the government that have a few basic pieces of equipment such as a scale and examining table, and materials such as gauze, syringes, and gloves. They are itinerantly staffed. Nurses or physicians from other clinics make infrequent rounds to these *casas de salud*, primarily using them for vaccination or other basic health campaigns. The *casa de salud* in Amatlán is hardly ever used because there are no medical personnel staffing it. It was built in 2002 with great fanfare (and partly funded with village money) and promised to improve people's health and increase their access to "development." When the *casa* was first built, the physician and nurse from Tepatepec came up to the village about once every four months to carry out check-ups and to ensure that people were following *autocuidado* by boiling their drinking water, sweeping their homes, and burning their trash. Everyone in the village was required to attend these visits, particularly women and children, though it seemed slightly redundant to do this inasmuch as the people already went regularly to the clinic. Over time these visits have dwindled to at most two visits a year. As Aurora, the kindergarten teacher, said caustically, "The *casa de salud* [was built] here, but well, it is hardly used at all." The building now mostly stands empty, a mark of government programs gone awry.

The Clinic in Ixhuatlán de Madero

This was the first government clinic built in this municipality. Situated just two blocks from the town's main civic-religious square, this clinic attends to people from over thirty surrounding villages. Though it is not a large clinic (with three physicians and four nurses and support staff), it attends to over a hundred people a day. Its centrality makes it an ideal location for people wishing to drop by the clinic if they happen to be in Ixhuatlán; this is especially the case on Sunday—market day.

Because historically this was the only local clinic available to people, it continues to retain that position in people's minds. Before the development of other clinics in the region, this was the only source of medical care. People had to make the arduous journey—along unpaved roads and across deep rivers—if they needed emergency medical care. Many of the people I spoke with continued to think of it as a second option if their own clinic happened to be closed or full. Some of the women of Amatlán had given birth there, because they went into labor when their regular clinic in Tepatepec was closed.

Doctora Felipa is the life and soul of the clinic. A stocky woman with short hair and a friendly, open smile that could quickly turn impatient, she was enthusiastic about my research. On the day we met, she proudly gave me a tour of the facility and insisted that I take photos of all the rooms. She sent the orderly to tidy and sort out the rooms to make them look as impeccable as possible. The delivery room is particularly striking in its medical starkness. The white tile floor blended into the stainless steel of the equipment, which consisted of a delivery table with metal stirrups, metal table and lamp, and steel slops bucket. An infant scale and examining console completed the equipment in the room. Though low-tech by many standards, it was still starkly medical and could be part of a clinic anywhere in the world. It was completely lacking in local color.

During my visits to the clinic, I would spend part of the time in the waiting room, chatting with the patients, and the rest of the time in the physician's office, observing the physician-patient interactions. Doctora Felipa would greet each female visitor, regardless of her purpose for being at the clinic, with "Are you carrying out family planning?" For most of the women, the answer was a cautious yes.

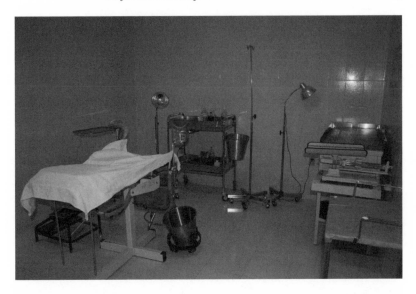

Figure 3.1. Birthing room in the Ixhuatlán clinic

Felipa's office contains an examining table, a desk covered in patients' files, some shelves with medications behind the desk, a scale, an X-ray viewer, and a sink. It is lit with a fluorescent light, which makes everything look very pale. The only color comes from the posters hanging on the wall. I usually sat on one of the two chairs available for patients. It was broken. Though the patients varied daily, the scene outside in the waiting room and within the office did not change much. In my field notes, one can see that the descriptions for each of my visits are quite similar. Through the open doorway, I could see the women outside waiting for their turn. The women waiting looked poorer than the ones I met in Amatlán and its surrounding villages. Many carry their infants in a *re-bozo*, a woven shawl. Some women feed their infants with bottles of milk. One woman is breastfeeding. The older kids look a little bit untidy, and their clothes are frayed. Many are eating cookies and other junk food.

Patients flowed in and out of the physician's office. Doctora Felipa had each patient's medical chart and would use that alongside a quick interview to diagnose the patient's sickness or condition and to decide what remedy to prescribe. Most consultations followed the same pattern. One of the patients, Narcisa, an older woman from the village of Jopala, came in with various complaints. She carried a woven bag over her shoulder and a plastic bag in her hands with her paperwork and some belongings. Speaking in a very low voice, she was almost inaudible. The physician began by asking her if she was enrolled in Seguro Popular to which she answered no, that she had been told to wait for news on when her family would eventually be enrolled in that program. [4] Felipa typed up notes as she consulted with her. Narcisa was forty-six years old. Doctora Felipa turned to me and said that she herself was forty-nine, but that the woman looked much older—more worn—than she did.

Narcisa said, "My bones hurt, my stomach hurts; I have gastritis, fever. It has been 15 days. I can't carry water. I have to get wood daily [and can't]." She added that she could not wash clothes, and that "the sun harms me. My head hurts." As she said this she coughed. Doctora Felipa told her to lie on the examining table with her head to the wall. She checked her eyes and mouth and told her that one of her teeth was not looking well and had to come out. She told her to go next door to the dentist. She then checked her heart with the stethoscope. After this, she told her to get up, and she sat back down at her desk to type up her diagnosis. She then turned to me and said, "She forcibly requires a programmed appointment because of Oportunidades. If the [women] don't come they get a black mark [against their name] in the program. What I do is to move their appointments along so that they don't come in vain and so they don't get a mark." She turned back to Narcisa and gave her folic acid pills, saying, "*Mija*,[5] take these three times a day." Then, giving her a prescription, she said, "For the pain, take these [others] once a day, which you can get at the pharmacy." The consultation took less than seven minutes.

The Clinic in Tepatepec

The clinic in Tepatepec opened its doors in 1999. Though it originally had a staff of seven, that number has dwindled to two and a half: the doctor Braulio; Juliana, the primary nurse; and Salvina, the nurse from the neighboring village of Huayacán, who works only a few irregular hours a month. Neither of the primary staff is from the region. Their ethnicity is *mestizo*, and they speak no indigenous language; they are from Poza Rica. Braulio drives both of them into the area on Monday morning, and they stay until Friday morning. They live in two rooms adjoining the clinic and eat their meals in a small eatery in Tepatepec. No one staffs the clinic on the weekend.

Six villages share this clinic. It is centrally located and relatively easy to reach, since it is on a highway leading from Llano de Enmedio to Ixhuatlán. It is a single-story concrete building with four small rooms and a small

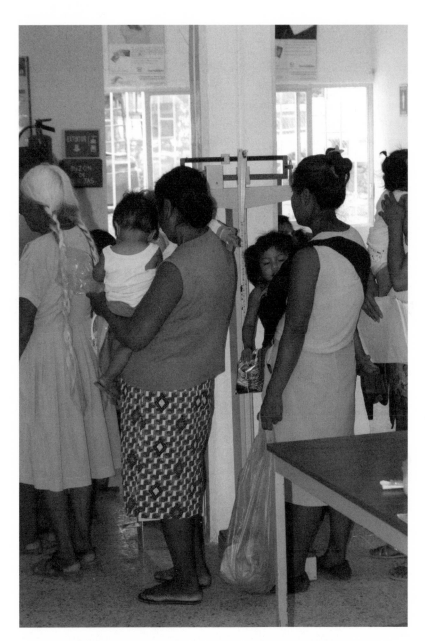

Figure 3.2. Waiting at the clinic

pharmacy. The pharmacy is a recent addition funded through the Seguro Popular program. The waiting room and nurse's station is on an outer veranda and is covered by a roof (which does not afford people much protection during inclement weather). There are some rough wooden benches and blue plastic chairs for people to sit on while they wait to be attended. The clinic sees approximately twenty-five people a day, whose average time spent waiting at the clinic is two hours.

Until 2004, going to the clinic entailed getting there early and waiting patiently for several hours for one's turn. The staff has recently implemented a new system of appointments, reminiscent of medical care elsewhere. This new system has made the physician's and nurse's lives easier, as they know who is expected to show up and whom to keep track of (though walk-ins are still accepted). And while it also helped the people to know when to go and to not have to wait so long to be attended, in many ways, it has also served to constrict their medical lives: their activities are more easily tracked, and any noncompliance is much more likely to be penalized.

The medical services offered by the clinic include such things as general check-ups, vaccinations, pediatric care, basic gynecological care, prevention of conditions such as diabetes and high blood pressure, and family planning. While Doctor Braulio and Nurse Juliana have good intentions and want to make sure that they treat the ills of their patients, there is some strain between them and their patients. The relationship between the clinicians and the patients is awkward at best. The groups come from very different backgrounds, and in these interactions, the differences rather than the similarities are emphasized. Juliana credits her efforts for what she views as the positive changes in people's health. She said proudly,

> In the past the women would arrive with such an *odor;* they bathed but I don't think they would scrub their bodies with a sponge. . . . It was difficult to get near some of them; their smell would make me feel sick. I think they would only splash water on themselves and did not bathe well. They say that people don't change, but they do change with a lot of effort [on our part].

The way she has managed to get people to follow *autocuidado* and assume responsibility for their health and well-being is by being strong and using a particularly forceful tone with the patients, "or they won't listen to me." And though she laughingly admitted that people found her grumpy and crotchety, she preferred it that way. She said she could continue to influence people's health with her strength.

The Hospital in Llano de Enmedio

The hospital in Llano de Enmedio was built in late 2004. It is a stunning building for this area and is purported to offer first-class service to the people of the region. Having become accustomed to the small-scale clinics of this region, I experienced some reverse culture shock at entering the hospital for the first time. It is at the end of a short cobbled road off the main street of Llano de Enmedio, which has a ragged collection of car repair shops, eateries, and miscellaneous stores. The salmon-colored structure appears mirage-like at the end of the cobbled road and gives the viewer the impression of having come across a private hospital in Arizona or Nevada, because of the desert color and vegetation scheme. As I entered through the glass doors, I realized that even the oppressive heat of the summer was left outside. The main waiting room had rows and rows of blue plastic chairs, only a couple of which were occupied. Ceiling fans lazily moved the air around, making the large, cavernous room quite comfortable. There seemed to be no medical staff visible, except Azalea, an administrator who was delighted to talk about the hospital and its services.

Providing its patients with more complete primary care than the clinics, the hospital is designed as a recipient of referrals from the outlying *centros de salud*. Most services are free or have a nominal cost, particularly for people who receive the Seguro Popular or are enrolled in Oportunidades.

The head nurse, Leonor, seemed very harassed most of the time; she hurriedly shared the hospital's policy on family planning. She repeatedly said, "The percentage [of women who are contracepting] is very low." She said the family-planning protocols come directly from the Ministry of Health in Poza Rica. The quota is meant to be 100 percent of women receiving family planning, but the hospital rates fall significantly below this; for the first three months of 2007, there were thirty-six obstetric events, and only eleven women accepted a semipermanent or permanent contraceptive method (30.5 percent). Leonor said that women have to provide a "signature that they don't accept a [contraceptive] method" so that there is a record of the hospital's promoting it and the women's refusing it. They manage first-stage family planning (condom and hormonal) as well as second-stage (IUDs, vasectomies, and tubal ligations). They kept good records of the contraceptive rates used as well as of the obstetric events. Their records showed that for 2006 and 2007 there were no vasectomies. In 2006, there were almost ten times as many women receiving IUD as tubal ligations, while in 2007, that proportion had dropped to just over four to one respectively. It is perhaps telling that the records use the Spanish verb *apear*—to depose or bring down something—to describe their efforts to convince women to contracept.

This hospital is classified as an "*hospital integral*" (whole- or integral-care hospital) and includes the primary-care practices of gynecology, general medicine, surgery, and pediatrics. These types of hospitals are run by the Mexican Ministry of Health and are located in smaller towns or villages, serving as support for small rural clinics. There are twelve beds in the hospital as well as two operating rooms, a delivery room, and several other rooms for emergency care. In addition, it offers laboratory services, X-rays, and a pharmacy. Its staff is meant to consist of a dozen physicians and double the number of nurses and support personnel. According to Doctor Gustavo, a general physician who looked to be barely out of medical school, they attend to between 100 and 120 births a year.

The hospital has struggled financially, however, and for more than a year after it was built it was not able to offer many services: the administrators lacked funds to fix the generator; they did not have all the equipment they needed; they were understaffed; and, most importantly, very few people came in for care. For the first few months, it was almost bereft of patients, and the staff tended to just sit around waiting expectantly for the arrival of a patient. During this time, there was only one general physician on site for emergencies and one dentist. There were five nurses. Approximately five more physicians (including a gynecologist and a pediatrician) were expected by October 2005. In 2007, the staff consisted of twenty nurses and five doctors.

By the time I left Amatlán in July 2007, only a handful of people from the village had ever attended the hospital; some of them went for an emergency (it is open twenty-four hours) or to have tests ordered by the physician at the clinic. When I asked the people if they ever went to the hospital instead of the clinic, most looked quizzical. They seemed unaware that they could go there and that the services were either inexpensive or free.

The reason for the lack of patients was political. This hospital was built against the wishes of many local activists, who had hoped it would be placed in the *sierra*, and serve more remote populations. Azalea, the hospital administrator, explained, slightly defensively, that there were few patients because "the communities have not been told that the hospital is here. Because those belonging to the PRD [a political party] protested against the hospital because they didn't want it here and that it would be better further away, by the river [Vinazco].[6] Well now that there is a new president he does not want to spread the word. And he is just waiting for there to be negative reports about the hospital." Doctor Gustavo echoed her words when he said that information about the role of the hospital "has not been disseminated." The use of the hospital as a political football is typical in Mexico of the way politicians build things to enhance their popularity without bothering to ensure that they are useful.[7] Because of this political stalemate, the hospital became a white elephant during its first few years.

Conflicted Relationships

Most of the women alluded to their conflicted relationship with the medical centers. On the one hand, they appreciated the free health care, especially during emergencies. But on the other hand, they struggled with the way they were treated and the tense relationship they had with the clinicians. What seemed apparent was that most of the women did not fully understand the benefits of preventative health care and *autocuidado*—which was the primary source of contention between them and the clinicians.

Local people's understanding of public health was not helped by some of the politically inspired programs organized by the Mexican Health Ministry. During the national vaccination week, the local clinics held various speech and photo events that were mandatory for the women participating in Oportunidades. The vaccination event in 2004 epitomized much of the confusion about the importance of public health. All the women from surrounding villages and their young children were expected to attend the vaccination week event held on a Saturday morning at the Tepatepec clinic. Several local VIPs and Health Ministry officials were in attendance, armed with pamphlets and cameras. After several, mostly self-congratulatory, speeches by the physician and a ministry health worker, one of the nurses held a young crying child on her lap and administered an oral vaccine as someone took photos. At the end of each speech and photo opportunity, the physician would pointedly mime clapping to encourage all the attendees to clap. Most of the women seemed to have little idea why they were there; they had simply been told that it was mandatory.

As part of the event, a parade up and down the main street of Tepatepec—where appropriate photos could be taken—was also expected. The local VIPs left after the speeches, which prompted the physician to ask the assembled women whether they wanted to parade or go back to Amatlán, where a soccer game between two rival villages was underway. Someone piped up, "Let's go to the game!" and the physician replied, "Okay, but let's pose for the photo as if we had just marched, now that [the VIPs] have left." He asked everyone to line up outside the clinic and hold up a banner that read "To vaccinate your children is to protect them for life." As the photo was taken, the VIPs drove up once more. Pretending that the aim all along had been to do the parade, the physician chivvied all of us attendees to walk. Chatting about how much sun was beating down on us, Lourdes and I joined the group. We walked by the main road, turned around at the end of the village, and walked back to the clinic. It took ten minutes. Once back at the clinic, the physician enthusiastically asked everyone to clap for the event and called the meeting to an end. The women quickly dispersed and began to walk back to Amatlán, hoping to catch the end of the soccer game.

The event was designed as a politico-bureaucratic function inaugurating the vaccination week. Though within some of the speeches and within the banner itself lay information about the importance of vaccination for children's health, most of this information was hidden under layers of political cosmetic language. At no point in the event were children vaccinated or was anything practical actually done. If the intent of these public health weeks was to stimulate self-care and bodily awareness, then they fell short. Certainly the women vaccinated their children, but they seemed to do so because they were told to rather than because they knew the benefits. Indeed, years later when the government launched a campaign to vaccinate the elderly against pneumococcal infection, the fear spread like wildfire that "if you turn 60 years [of age] they will vaccinate you so that you will die. . . . That they are already too old." Perhaps if greater context and information were provided about the reason behind the vaccines, such misinformation would be avoided.

Fátima felt particularly disenchanted with the medical care at the clinic. Treating most of her family's illnesses at home, she rationalized it by stating, "Now with that clinic there are more illnesses than in the past. With more clinics, there are more illnesses." While no one else had this unusual opinion of the correlation between medical care and ill health, concern frequently revolved around the quality of health-care delivery. Adrian, Esperanza's son, was frequently sick with skin lesions, which he had tried to treat by lathering commercial crop pesticides onto his skin. This left him with enormous pustules and scars across his arms. He thus often went to the clinic in the hope of receiving some topical medication to alleviate his disfigurement. One morning, he returned furious, saying that he waited for hours but no clinician had ever appeared. He muttered, "The [physician] does not do his duty."

The concern with people's public health is central to Oportunidades and to the precepts of the small clinics serving the beneficiary families. The quality of people's drinking water was of much concern to Nurse Juliana. She bemoaned the pollution of the stream flowing through several of the villages, which was used for everything from washing people, dishes, and clothes to cleaning offal and rinsing out pesticide containers. She stated, with much concern,

> They are told not to bathe there, because then they show up [at the clinic] with lots of scabies, with diarrhea. And they are told to boil the water. Because those who aren't used to it then fall sick with diarrhea if they drink water that has not been boiled. But it is difficult to keep a watch on them, as I am not there. Whenever I visit [their homes] I ask them for water. And you can tell right away if it is not boiled, and so I say something to them. They told us [at the ministry] that they would send us a [health] promoter who would see to all this and would go to the communities to provide health development [information], and to give *pláticas*, and all [that]. But they have not sent her. I have to do it all myself. I function as a nurse, [a] promoter, I give the *pláticas*. But then the [women] come, they hear the *plática* and then go and tell the other women something else. And then they believe her. So I tell them, 'if you won't believe me, maybe that woman should give the *plática*.'

Evident from the words above is the conflict between notions of national public health—vaccination, potable water, or general health—and local people's misunderstandings of the reasons for the changes. The ambiguities existent between these conceptions led to an uncompromising redoubled effort at reeducating the people about preventative health care and its importance, while simultaneously disempowering this precise population through increasingly technical and medicalized public health schemes.

Forcing the Population Mission

In this region, there has been increasing erosion of local medical knowledge in general and women's knowledge in particular because of development and medical changes. Development and medicine are both forceful practices and powerful ideologies and have great influence on how women are thought of and how they think of their bodies. Within medicine, there are issues of power and dominance wherein the authority of the clinicians and institutions frequently constrain women's choices. For the women of this region, knowledge about their bodies in regard to medicine is "inextricably related to medical hegemony and social class" (Lazarus 1997:132). Because their bodies are controlled by development and medicine, they are gradually losing agentive control over them, particularly in the realm of reproductive choices. At present, though the women have seen a marked increase in their basic health, it has come at the expense of their ability to choose. A situation of intended authority emerges—one that develops from the country's history of *indigenismo* and modernity—and it is this authority to which the local women are responding.[8] This nexus creates the circumstances and processes that suggest a "forcible" undercurrent in these women's experiences within the medical setting.

All the clinicians I spoke with were unequivocally concerned with women having many children and the effects this could have on their lifestyle. Consequently, they implemented the Mexican national family-planning program with great zeal. They saw their role as facilitators of women's reproduction and used their power and authority to make their patients "see" the light. One of the physicians stated,

> The [women] are forced to come. [The frequency] depends on whether it's an adult then they come . . . once a year. If she's pregnant she's obligated to have at least seven [prenatal] consultations throughout her pregnancy. If she's carrying out family planning she is obligated to come each time she has an appointment according to her family planning method. If it's a child under five he's obligated to come to the nutritional management, which depends upon his nutritional status. If he's a normal child then he comes every six months. A normal child under one year comes five times before his first birthday. If the child is slightly malnourished then we see him monthly. If he is moderately malnourished then every fifteen days. If he is gravely or severely malnourished then we refer him to the hospital . . . for a pediatric situation of that sort.

For the women with whom I spoke, the term *forcible* carries a particular connotation wherein they do not have to be physically threatened to consider certain medical procedures forced. The process is much more insidious than simply overt threats or force. These women interact on a regular basis with medical staff in clinics and hospitals where their knowledge about health and their bodies carries less weight than the knowledge of the clinicians. In these contexts, their knowledge becomes discredited and devalued in favor of the authoritative knowledge of physicians and nurses (Maternowska 2006). Specifically, given the supervisory role granted to the clinicians by Oportunidades, including the authority to report a woman who is not complying with the conditions, most women feel they must follow the orders at the clinic, even if the conditions of Oportunidades are not being violated. There are powerful sanctions (perceived or actual) at play here if a patient does not comply with the directives of the clinic. As Juliana, the nurse in Tepatepec, said to me one day, "If we mark them as absent their support from [Oportunidades] is taken away. We have them nicely bound [to this system]."[9]

Consequently, when a physician or nurse tells them that they should undergo certain medical procedures, the women would consider these procedures forced because the idea that they had real choices in this context is absurd (Overmyer-Velázquez 2003).

Compliance with the physician's or nurse's orders in the clinical context is viewed as a mark of a developed and modern person. And with the onus of responsibility placed squarely on the mothers for building up the future of the Mexican state, compliance becomes of even greater importance. In the majority of the encounters I witnessed, there was an undercurrent of concern about mothers' compliance, or perceived lack thereof. The staff overlooked the social or economic distress felt by their patients. As Catherine Maternowska (2006:78) shows in her work on a family-planning clinic in one of the poorest slums of Port-au-Prince, Haiti, there are various reasons for lack of compliance that "transcend traditional public health parameters." These encounters frequently elicit a technical and medical response to women's health issues, which, as Maternowska observes in Haiti and Nancy Scheper-Hughes (1993) observes in Brazil, are easier than actually confronting the social and structural factors and realities that women face. Rarely did clinicians allow leeway for alternative options or someone's personal solutions. Initiative—or constrained choice—was never seen as such; instead such people were always viewed as lazy, ignorant, disobedient, or bad patients. At the end of a long day of seeing patients, one of the physicians turned to me and, sighing, said, "It's just that they don't want to advance; they are this way because they want to. . . . The [women] just stay at home, marginalized, and have kids."

Even in contexts where the physician was clearly wrong, somehow the patients were painted as the problem for preventing the population mission from being properly implemented. Salomé, a twenty-year-old woman wearing a long black skirt and green blouse came into the Ixhuatlán clinic with her three-and-a-half-month-old baby in June 2007. The physician turned to me and said in a proud voice, "She is contracepting." Salomé immediately replied, "[No, I am not], not since you told me that you would find an IUD for me. I don't want pills or injections. My husband does not want to use condoms." In the awkward pause that followed, the physician rephrased her statement, saying that she only had small IUDs that would fall out without Salomé noticing, thus risking becoming pregnant. Adroitly turning the tables on Salomé—blaming her large uterus on her inability to have proper contraception—she told her to fetch her husband from the waiting room so she could drum some sense into him. He was a young man wearing trendy clothes who walked in carrying his toddler daughter in his arms. The physician began scolding him about the importance of contraception saying, "You have three children and you are only 20 years old."

Salomé sat quietly in the chair with her face downcast and a very embarrassed smile on her face. Her husband stood shyly, and slightly sullenly, with his arm on his waist, swinging a piece of paper, giving the impression he did not care. After the physician had harangued him for a while in a harsh tone to get his attention, the husband admitted that he did not know how to use condoms. The physician tutted and said that she would show him. But a search through the office did not reveal any condoms. So she tried to explain to him verbally how it should be unrolled onto the penis and taken off after sexual intercourse. Salomé appeared even more embarrassed than before, never once looking up. Her stiff, hunched shoulders revealed her discomfort. The physician eventually gave up and called the male nurse. When the nurse came in, she asked him if he had a condom, which he produced from his wallet. So, with condom in hand, the physician unrolled it onto her fingers and showed Salomé's husband how to use it. He continued to stand awkwardly, but the physician took his silence as acquiescence and soon dismissed them. When they left, the physician gave me a knowing glance and rolled her eyes at what she perceived as the stubbornness of her patients.

Salomé's case is not unique, as many female patients with potential for high fertility are treated as willfully stubborn and as incapable of making sensible decisions about their reproductive lives. Maternowska (2006) points to this exact situation in her work on a fertility clinic in Haiti, where women were contemptuously classified as irresponsible even before they set foot in the clinic. Even though Salomé clearly wanted access to contraception—she would be the classic statistic of the "unsatisfied demand" mentioned by Tuirán et al. (2002)—her own body betrays her and is used against her. She has a large uterus because she has already given birth to three children, but because of its size she will not be able to receive an IUD that would prevent her having any more children. This would lead to her uterus becoming "baggier and baggier" as Juliana's words in the book's

Introduction show. Salomé is not allowed to "let [her uterus] rest" because she is "constantly using it."

What Salomé's case shows is that rather than noncompliance or stubbornness, it was actually a structural situation that created the high number of children she already had at the age of twenty. Within this structure one finds (1) a husband's refusal to acknowledge his ignorance about condoms—such an admittance would emasculate him, (2) a low stock of appropriate family-planning devices (IUDs and condoms) for needy patients, and (3) a miscommunication regarding sexuality and reproduction between the physician and the patient. In Salomé's situation, even though both women are intent on a similar goal (contracepting), their interpretation of the issue leaves them at odds with each other. Though I never saw Salomé again—she was from one of the remote communities served by the Ixhuatlán clinic—I would hazard a guess that the rushed explanation of condom usage would not be enough to guarantee her husband's adherence. And unless the next time she came in there was a stock of appropriately sized IUDs, it is likely that she would soon be pregnant with her fourth child.

The Male Mindset: The Partner's Role in Shaping Motherhood

Men can play an important role in women's choices about reproduction (Browner 2000), because women will often incorporate the wishes of their male partners into their own reproductive activities, sometimes even sublimating their own desires to those of their spouses (Nazar Beutelspacher et al. 2003). The women I spoke with fall into five categories with regard to their husband's role in contraception: (1) those who did not want to contracept but underwent a semipermanent or permanent method per their husband's wishes; (2) those who did not contracept per their husband's wishes, even if that was not what the women wanted; (3) those who decided to contracept (either overtly or covertly) despite their husband's opinions; (4) those who chose not to contracept despite their husband's wishes to the contrary; and (5) those who reached the decision to contracept together with their husbands. I became especially interested in the ways that the national family-planning mission espoused by the physicians and nurses interplayed with the men's wishes and concerns.

Husbands frequently shape and reduce women's control over their reproduction, which is compounded by the paternalism present in the medical setting. Benita's story shows the synergy present between her husband's wishes and those of the clinic:

Yes, I was operated. . . . My husband told me that the nurse said we had to be operated, to sign up [for the operation]. To be operated already. My husband says "go to sign up" but I am scared. But I went to sign up, and he says he will sign [the consent form]. . . ." Better to not have any more kids," he says. "You did not have a girl, so that's it."

Her choice is constrained through her marital circumstances and is not unique (Nazar Beutelspacher et al. 2003). Indeed, her sister-in-law Frida also was operated on per her husband's wishes. These women are married to brothers who are very patriarchal and who have taken strict control over their wives' reproductive bodies. Neither woman felt she had any choice in reproductive matters. It was these women's husbands' desires that determined their lack of choice, which was facilitated through the contraceptive mission of the clinic. Adela's reproductive life also included her husband's input, but she saw it more as a negotiation than an imposition; yet she acknowledged that men's wishes determined most women's choices. She said,

You must look after [yourself]. You have to be in agreement with your husband. . . . I see many getting an operation. But not I; I feel I am fine as I am. . . . The doctor gets angry because the [women] get pregnant and they have four or five [children]. He says that three is enough. But if the husband says no, then the woman can't say anything. Whatever the man wants.

Though the consent process of the clinic requires that both husband and wife sign the form, there is likely little understanding at the clinic of each particular patient's domestic relationship, and the means by which a decision has been reached. Though women in this region experience relatively high gender equality, many larger decisions are frequently made by the men. This situation is ignored or misunderstood by the clinicians, who assume that the signing of the consent form is an indication of agreement.

Benita's and Frida's situation is actually quite unusual. In reality, the reverse is most often true; several of the husbands of the women I spoke with refused their wives permission to use contraceptives or be sterilized. Alicia mentioned her husband's refusal to allow her to be sterilized; she said, "[The doctor] doesn't want women to have children, he wants them all to be sterilized. He wanted me to be sterilized but my husband didn't want me to. He said that God gave me my body intact and that I shouldn't do that. He didn't let me be operated." One of the nurses also commented on this situation and said, "Because of machismo the men do not want [contraception]; they say that [they'll have] as many [children] as God wants, but they go too far because they have too many."

Doctora Felipa in Ixhuatlán placed much blame for the lack of family planning on the men. At one point she saw that her next patient was a man and said to me, as the man walked in, "If you want to know the mindset of the men, here it is." Many of the mothers I spoke with stated frequently that their spouses had a significant amount of control over their reproductive bodies. The medical personnel were often extremely exasperated with the men in this regard and held them directly responsible for the large families in the region. Doctora Felipa put it bluntly: "Here the man is the one with worth. Why? Because he's the one who goes to the fields. From the time they are little they go to the fields. Not the girl; she will get married." In the staffs' minds, the wiliness and stubbornness of the female patients was matched only by the utter willfulness and macho attitude of the men, who were perceived to simply want more children to control their wives' bodies and increase their sense of manhood. Beatriz, a young nurse in the hospital in Llano de Enmedio, said to me, "Many people still exist who are [this way] . . . in fact, the men I see are very *machista*. [They say], 'No one will keep you, I keep you; you will have the [number of] children I want.' All those things happen here."

While this chauvinist attitude was much less normative than believed by the clinicians, there is no denying that many women are forced by their husbands to have a certain number of children. The *pláticas* of Oportunidades often addressed these issues alongside information about family planning and the proper family size. But until the *pláticas* are aimed at both men and women, the situation is unlikely to change much. The women are simply armed with more information, but with no practical means of changing their husbands' behaviors. Men's wishes are taken into consideration in this process, which frequently is contrary to the "external institutional structures and ideologies intended to make it possible for women to limit their fertility" (Browner 2000:779). It is a situation where a woman has to balance her own wishes for family size, her husband's, her income from Oportunidades, and the national population mission espoused at the clinics and hospitals encouraging a reduction in her fertility.

"Paying me the respect I deserve": Nurses' Role in Mothers' Health

The clinicians at the medical centers promote family planning every time a woman comes in, even if her health issue during those visits is unrelated to reproduction. Mothers are met at the start of their consultation with the question "Are you contracepting?" As one of the nurses stated: "We have the duty to inform them about contraception every time they come in, because the greatest benefit [of contraception] is to have a better quality of life." She added, "We do not force them [to contracept] because it is a free decision. We simply insist again, until the woman finally wishes to [contracept]."

When the women go to the clinic or hospital, they interact most frequently with the nurse. The nurse is the first person they talk to and who checks their vital signs; she has their files and fills them out, and she asks about their home life. She also makes suggestions about lifestyle changes, additional treatments, and follow-ups, since she is also the last person whom they talk to before they leave. The nurse's most important role is regarding Oportunidades, since she is also the person who marks their attendance on the program's roster, making her role pivotal in women's compliance. This makes nurses' role much more important in the women's health than just as support staff for physicians. Though physicians are considered to be the ones who are in charge and who make the important decisions, nurses also influence the women's lives because they interact with the women to a much greater extent than the physicians do. Juliana saw her influence on her patients' health emerge through her own strength. She said, "I have to speak to them in a firmer tone of voice, rather than the low one we are talking in right now. It's just that if I talk to them in a low [voice] I see that they pay no attention and they don't pay me the respect that I deserve. That is why I talk to them firmly. I decided that from the start." It is through their position of authority as clinicians and gatekeepers for Oportunidades that nurses are central to the process by which the women become informed about their reproductive bodies and the eventual decisions they take regarding them.

It is evident that the women's ability to make choices about their reproductive bodies is constrained by the link between Oportunidades and medicine. The nurses, as clinicians who monitor the women's compliance with Oportunidades, use their authority to persuade the patients to use birth control and undergo sterilization. These nurses are key models in the web of development programs to lead to a modern Mexico. Matilde, the mother of four young children, pointed out to me as she prepared lunch, "The doctor gets angry and tells the [women] to be sterilized; [he says] that we shouldn't have more children. The nurse gets very angry and she even shouts. She doesn't like there to be so many [at the clinic]." Esperanza told me later,

> If one does not go to the appointment they take away [Oportuni-dades;] . . . that is why you always see those women who have lots of children going every day [to the clinic]. . . . The women have to go or they take away their [Oportunidades]. Their file would be unsigned [they have to sign to indicate their attendance] and then if someone checks and it is empty they take away her [Oportunidades].

In these settings, the nurses are perceived as the keepers of knowledge, resources, and technology about the reproductive body and therefore capable and authorized to influence and even make decisions about the women's bodies. Their authority effectually disempowers the women about their own bodies and decisions regarding them. Also, because the women depend on the money from Oportunidades, they find themselves having to follow the conditions set by the program. As Juana stated: "And one has to go because if one doesn't get to the appointment one is scolded at the clinic. Yes, they just scold us, they scold us a lot." Since the medical centers in this region are intimately tied to Oportunidades and the staff has the authority to report any woman who is not complying with these conditions, the women feel they have to follow the treatment options for fear of losing their monetary aid.

Nurses took their role of managers of the mothers' connection to Oportunidades very seriously. They felt it was their duty to correct problematic behaviors—such as missing appointments. Juliana often found herself scolding problematic patients. On one occasion, she scolded a group of mothers who had missed appointments, saying, "I tell you the requirements, so don't you complain if they take away your [monetary] support. Remember that you are the ones that take away your own support." On another occasion, she explained her role in managing women's health and attendance:

> I do mark them as absent. They are therefore forced to keep on coming, if not they would not come. I tell them that I will mark them as absent, and I follow through. Those who have more than two or three absences are automatically removed from [Oportunidades]. It is noted in their file. I always let them know so it does not come as a surprise. Though it is not my obligation [to do so] I do [warn] them.

Nurse Gilda, at the clinic in Ixhuatlán, stated that once their money is taken away, the women "are not given another chance because their [noncompliance] shows that they are irresponsible and not interested. Every two months a report is sent to see if they are complying." For some women, being removed from Oportunidades did come as a surprise, however, such as for the following woman, who expressed her concern while in Doctora Felipa's office: "They removed me, I don't know [why]. . . . I brought my son in every month [to the clinic], but they would not pass me inside [to see the doctor]. And the [other] *doctora* told me that I was no longer in Oportunidades. And I would bring him every month, every month to see her." While the clinicians use Oportunidades as a tool to obtain women's compliance, their intent is not malicious. Instead, the connection between clinics and the program is something that is convenient, enabling them to treat the health conditions of their patients and implement their contraceptive mission. It is within these interactions between the mothers and the clinicians that the friction and complexities intrinsic in their interactions emerge, especially in light of the entangled nature of the clinical setting and Oportunidades.

Significant unintended consequences emerge when Oportunidades is implemented, monitored, and managed by the linked groups—the clinics and hospitals. Because these linked groups are also acting under the rubric of the national population policies, one finds that both Oportunidades and the country's population mission become coalesced in the clinics and hospitals and directed at the target population of indigenous, rural woman. The physicians control access to Oportunidades as well as to actual health care, making them doubly powerful in this context—they unintentionally become agents of the development program. Additionally, confusion about health care and health knowledge arises out of this situation—often disempowering the women and their families in the process.

Because the mothers are not interested in risking an important part of their income, they comply with the attendance as well as with many of the procedures offered at the health centers. The mothers view the connection between Oportunidades and the clinics as so strong that they would be unable to differentiate between the elements of Oportunidades that they must follow and those that simply emerge from the synergy with the clinic. The outcome of this situation is that powerful people control women's financial lives and consequently also control their reproductive lives.

CHAPTER 4

Expectations of Good Motherhood

"Motherhood is the most highly judged state of your life." This was said to me by one of my friends in the United States during the early days of my pregnancy, a few years after I returned from Amatlán. In this state, my friend—who is the mother of three children, two of whom are twins—said, people will judge you and correct you and punish you for any behavior that is seen to be a transgression of the acceptable norms of society. Motherhood is equally observed and disciplined in the global South among economically disadvantaged populations—yet the surveillance and discipline come not only from one's peers, but also from government bodies and actors who can mete out significant punishment for transgressions. Criticism from one's peers, while perhaps not pleasant, is rarely a threat to one's livelihood and survival. For middle- and upper-class women, modernity is about choices, whereas for indigenous women, it is about submitting to control.

"People have become more aware": Motherhood under Surveillance

The success of Oportunidades comes not only from the top-down directives and outright threats tied to compliance, but also in its creation of biopower among the beneficiary women. Biopower is the way by which power is manifested through people's daily practices, through which people "engage in self-surveillance and self-discipline," thereby subjugating themselves (Pylypa 1998:21). As Ewald (1986:8) states, through biopower the state has the responsibility to ensure that its population behaves in the "most prophylactic manner possible." Women's bodies, as entry and exit points of danger, become regulated through overt forms of power, where their habits, health and hygiene, or reproduction and sexuality become paramount for modern nation states intent on protecting the life of its population.

Individuals are created through their categorization by those in power—these individuals are given a particular identity that is tied up with certain assumptions and norms that the individual is expected to follow and fulfill. For instance, Jacqueline, Emma's teenage daughter, stated, "People have become more aware.[1] . . . Well, in the past they were ignorant. If someone from outside came by they would rapidly manipulate them." In this way, the individual becomes a subject who is, as Foucault would put it, "subservient to someone else by control and dependence, and tied to [her] own identity by a conscience or self-knowledge" (Wetterberg 2004:29). Subservience and dependence are maintained through surveillance and punishment. Surveillance is a particularly effective form of control as it is constant, quiet, all-seeing, and all-inclusive (Wetterberg 2004:29). There is no specific time or place for surveillance, but rather people can observe others—and be observed in turn—while they carry out their daily lives. They are "perpetually supervised" (Foucault 1995:176–77). Cristina echoed this precise thought when she said, "If you don't [keep your home clean], they report you. The women of Oportunidades come and check that everything is clean. And you might think that that's it, but no, there is always someone watching."

This type of surveillance in itself is not negative, but it does demonstrate how informed people are of each other's movements and activities. It additionally contributes to women being able to consciously monitor (and criticize) each other's spending of the Oportunidades money. This monitoring tended to flare up just after the authorities had handed out the money. Women would line up to take a truck down to either of the market towns, ready to buy the necessities for their families. But there were always certain women who were criticized for spending their money on things that were not considered necessities and for just buying luxuries. These women became targets of idle gossip about their mothering abilities. Most of these women were those who received more money than the others—because they had more children or their children were either female or older or both—and so this incited jealousy.

This concern with the biopolitics of the body, in this case women's bodies, emphasizes what Foucault would call the "comprehensive measures, statistical assessments and interventions" that are aimed at the body politic (Hacking 1991:183). These ideas were taken by the emerging Mexican nation in the early twentieth century and developed into a strict surveillance and control of the problematic populations, especially the women's

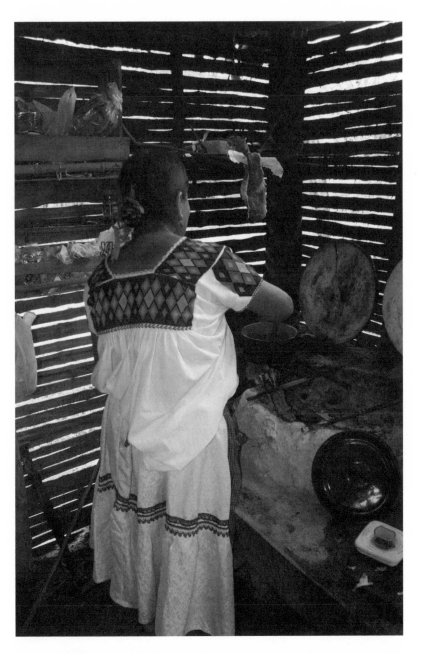

Figure 4.1. A kitchen in Amatlán

capacities to reproduce. Surveillance in Amatlán comes both from those of equal standing and from those of higher rank. Women supervise and keep each other under surveillance on a daily basis. Women spend much of their day in the kitchen, preparing food and cleaning up. The walls of most kitchens are made of vertical wood poles that often have quite large gaps between them, as well as a large space between them and the thatched or corrugated roof, to allow smoke to escape. This architecture has the added bonus of allowing women to see the activity outside their home-stead and to keep track of who is doing what and where they are going.

I found it puzzling the first few weeks of my time in the village when I would tell Esperanza that I was on my way to visit someone on the other side of the village and she would tell me that I was wasting my time as that person had gone to town, was washing clothes, or had gone to visit a sick relative. She always seemed to know where people were at all times, despite not having left the house. Much of this knowledge is circulated around the village through the informational greeting system—where people tell each other as they walk around the village where they are going and what they will do there. Yet a large part of it comes from looking out and observ-ing what the neighbors are doing. Spending so much time in Esperanza's kitchen, chatting over a delicious cup of sweetened coffee and home-baked breads, I became equally adept at craning my neck at the slightest indica-tion of movement on the road along her house.

The women would often use the official gatherings at the *Casa de Salud* to air grievances. These meetings have the added function of extending surveillance to each other through the exchange of gossip and other in-formation. During one of these mothers' meetings, many of the women arrived late. Those who had arrived on time began grumbling at the late-ness. Some of them began to round on the absent Frida, who was seen as a troublemaker. Genoveva, who was always very vocal in her criticism, said loudly, "Well, if these [women] don't come they should be marked as ab-sent." Nodding, many women agreed, stating that then it would be obvious to the Oportunidades authorities that the absent women were not follow-ing orders. These meetings thus had the function of airing the problems certain women would have with others not following the rules ordered by Oportunidades. There was an effort at resolution, which frequently took the form of small fines to be paid by the transgressor.

The women are also under surveillance by the teachers at the school and by the staff at the Tepatepec clinic. This form of surveillance is much more active than the one carried out by the women in their daily lives, but

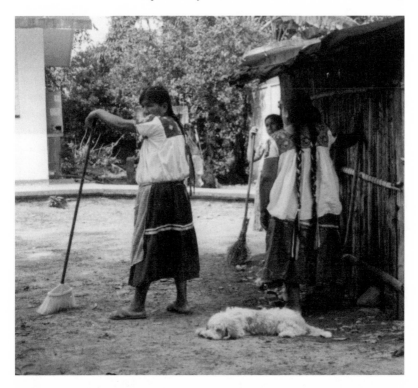

Figure 4.2. Women resting in the shade prior to a meeting

it is insidious because it taps into these surveillance networks and uses the information gathered to control and punish women who do not conform. Both the *promotora* and the *auxiliar* act as go-betweens for the surveillance of the women, particularly at the clinical setting. Both women went to the clinic on a regular basis to receive instructions for themselves as well as to convey messages and instructions to the enrolled women. Esperanza was particularly critical of the connection between the clinic and the female authorities. She bitterly said one day,

> If we do not go, [the doctor] scolds us and takes away our [Oportunidades]. He told the *auxiliar* and the *promotora* that if we don't go to a meeting [they should] mark us as absent and to leave the [space where we have to sign our attendance] blank. And for them not to say anything [about this] to us but to give our name to the doctor and that he will make sure that the [Oportunidades] is taken away.

She then proceeded to tell me a couple of anecdotes about female neighbors whose money was reduced after they did not attend a regular meeting with the physician. She added, "Yes, the doctor tells us that if we do not comply our [Oportunidades] will be taken away." Much of this relationship between the mothers and the clinicians is reminiscent of Allen's (2002) findings among women in Tanzania, where the implementation of the Safe Motherhood Initiative was designed to be supportive of women's prenatal care yet resulted in punishments for perceived noncompliance with the tenets of the medical system.

Intertwined with the women's personal duties to the Oportunidades rules are expectations of community participation in the aesthetic appearance of the clinic. An alternating group of women organized by the female authorities from the various surrounding villages were expected to come to the clinic and sweep the floors and keep the vegetation in front tidy. Esperanza said to this, "The doctor tells the *promotora* [to tell us to go]. [And if we don't go] they also take away our [Oportunidades]. That is why we always have to go to the meetings and then to the doctor's *pláticas*, if not we get marked as absent."

Besides the monitoring the women receive from their peers and authorities, they are also threatened with being marked as transgressors and removed from the program. The simple threat of removal is enough to gain women's compliance, given their concerns for their children's welfare. As Foucault (1991) suggests, the fact that the women have transgressed is perceived by all as an illustration of some sort of failing in the wrongdoer, rather than a problem with the system itself.

The women of Amatlán are constantly measured and compared to one another, and as Wetterberg (2004) shows in her work on reproduction in the United States, they are made into a hierarchy based on the extent to which they follow these norms. So the women who follow the norms will be "good" women and mothers, while those further away from the norm and at the lower end of the hierarchy would be the "bad" women, the "bad" and problematic mothers, who disobey norms and rules.

Pláticas: *Getting a Talking To*

The *pláticas* are a very effective way for clinicians to impart information to their patients, as the women are required to participate or risk a black mark against their name. In these talks, the women receive advice on *auto-cuidado*—self-care—particularly about nutrition for themselves and their children, ways to improve their health, how to reduce health risks (by having regular check-ups, receiving prenatal care, detecting malnutrition, and so on), how to recognize symptoms of illness, how to treat certain basic illnesses (such as through oral rehydration therapy for diarrhea), how to use nutritional supplements for at-risk populations (pregnant women and infants), and how to keep their homes and environment clean, as well as information about contraception and family planning. The implementers of Oportunidades consider these *pláticas* to be a way for the individuals and the community to actively participate in their health care and a way to promote a "culture of preventive care," thereby empowering the individuals and communities involved (Skoufias 2005:6).

Manuel, the health promoter at the clinic in Ixhuatlán, was in charge of all the *pláticas* and all the Oportunidades and health-related issues for the municipality. He was a recent arrival to the area in 2007, being originally from the state capital of Xalapa, and had worked as the local health promoter for six years in the town of Papantla, several kilometers south of Poza Rica. He lived full time in Poza Rica and commuted daily to Ixhuatlán. He was very concerned about helping the women to become better mothers. He advocated for early initiation of breastfeeding and *estimulación temprana*—early stimulation of children's cognitive and intellectual development. He said that in the *pláticas* he would encourage mothers to stimulate their babies by talking to them and to "not always have the baby flat on its back on the floor." While he spoke kindly about the women enrolled in Oportunidades, he emphasized that this area was very underdeveloped and there were many customs and traditions that impeded development.

Cristina, Emma's eldest daughter, who has five children, two under the age of ten, cheerfully said to me after she came back from a *plática* in Tepatepec,

> I always like those *pláticas* because they tell us interesting things. There are many [women] who do not put into practice the things that the nurse tells us, but I do. They told us that there are some small organs in the stomach called *soldaditos* (little soldiers) and they help us to not get sick. . . . They also told us at what age we should marry because there is a village called La Huerta where the girls are getting married and having children at 14 or 15 [years of age]. And the doctor says that here in Amatlán that almost doesn't happen, that maybe earliest at 17, but that [over] there they are still just kids. That they should marry later.

She added that she learned a lot from these sessions, especially about nutrition and what to feed her children. She especially liked the ideas about nutrition as her youngest daughter, who was only five years old in 2004, had little interest in food. Every time we visited in her kitchen, Cristina would share her woes about feeding Clara. She said one morning, as she cooked tortillas for her children's luncheon,

> Oh, I don't know what to do with her. She doesn't want to eat. At nine months old she suddenly didn't want to eat and it was with great difficulty that I would get her to eat. She weighs less than she should at her age. The doctor is always checking her and he has de-wormed her various times and he has given her different vitamins, like Kiddie, but she still does not eat. . . . I have tried everything. But I have no money to take her to Álamo to a specialist, a pediatrician. She doesn't even want her milk. I have tried her with Nido, with Papilla Leche, with Chocomilk, Cal-C-Tose,[2] but she wants none of them. She only wants water-based Jell-O, but those don't give her nutrition. I no longer let her eat sweets or anything, because if not she eats even less. I don't know what to do!

When her children came into the kitchen, she fed them warm tortillas, egg, and salsa. She gave Clara a carefully and lovingly made *taco de huevo*— a tortilla filled with scrambled egg—which the little girl ate dispassionately, leaving most of it untouched. Cristina looked at me sadly and said, "She is always sick because her defenses are low because she does not eat. She is always sick." She felt comforted by the information shared at the *pláticas*, as they addressed the problem she had in feeding her daughter. She said, "They also told us not to drink so much soda, because we always try to find a way to buy it. But that it harms us. That it is better to have fruit juice. They also told us what foods were good and which ones not, and how to eat a balanced [diet]." The fact that she had just served me a large glass of red Kool-Aid in lieu of soda led me to think she interpreted the sugary packets to be the fruit juice of the nurse's words.

It was evident that some of the information imparted at the *pláticas* made little cultural sense. Esperanza recalled the same *plática* mentioned by Cristina, and she said that the nurse told them "not to eat [red] meat anymore." When I asked why, she answered, "She said that we should not eat it; that instead [we should eat] beans and potatoes and other [things], because [red] meat is bad if one eats too much. That it is harmful because it has too much fat and it damages the heart." While such a concern might make sense in an industrialized setting where eating red meat is normative, very few of the families in the region eat beef more than once or twice a month. Such a statement is confusing to the people, as it addresses a problem that does not actually exist and instead removes an important source of iron and protein from people's diets. So while reducing consumption of soda was an important goal—the Pepsi truck seemed to be the only vehicle that made its way into the village every Wednesday come rain or shine—the issue needed to be better addressed culturally for the people, because removing sodas but replacing them with Kool-Aid "fruit juices" was no better. And removing red meat from the diet in a one-size-fits-all fashion made little sense to people for whom meat was already a luxury.

Constructing Mothers: Stories of Amatlán's Women

The Good Mother

Most women in Amatlán consider themselves, their neighbors, and their friends to be good mothers. Almost all the women in the community labor in the domestic sphere—they cook the food, wash the clothes, and generally look after the house and children. Making *lonches*—lunches for the men in the fields and for the school-age children—is an integral part of their mothering. A good mother frets about what she is feeding her children. Though the terms the women use to talk about each others' mothering are similar to the good-bad dichotomy used by the mainstream, their interpretations and the reasons behind their interpretations are more nuanced. For the state, good mothers follow the rules, have few children, and invest in them emotionally; they are also expected to live in a nuclear family. For the women I met, good motherhood entailed a significant amount of investment, but also drawing from one's extended-kin network to achieve a child's success; *abuelas* and *ahuis* (grandmothers and aunts) were frequently key to the socialization process of any child.

Gloria, one of the poorest women in the village, constantly strove to make ends meet and feed her children. Despite her poverty, Gloria always has a gap-toothed and mischievous smile on her face and is always cheerful and talkative. She is in her late thirties and has five children, two of whom are twins. She is also very assertive, speaking her mind and questioning things that trouble or bother her. A few years earlier, one of her daughters passed away. She said, "She never spoke. She just used gestures. And she would just sit [inside the house]. And well, one day she died. She was nine years old." Her husband was particularly affected by their daughter's death, losing his faith and no longer attending the Pentecostal worship. Gloria stated that he had never been the same since. His grief has caused him to be frequently ill; it is embodied in his diminished and lost countenance, the hesitant way he speaks, and his inability to work regularly. Living next door to her parents, Gloria relied on them for daily help with her children or financial and emotional support. And while she and her sister-in-law, who lived in the same compound, were regularly engaged in disputes, they also depended on each other for childcare and household help. Gloria said regarding her family,

> Children are very troublesome. Mine always pester me to give them a coin to buy *tostes* and sweets.[3] We have very little money; my husband earns 80 pesos a day working [as a peon] in the *milpa*.[4] . . . I don't know [if I'll have any more children]. I already have five, but maybe the sixth will arrive. I don't want to be sterilized and my husband also does not want me to have an operation. I am frightened. And then they say that the doctors sell the stuff they remove. Who knows!?

Relying on condoms for family planning, she grumbled when the clinic ran out of them, and she had to be inventive to keep her husband away from her somehow. She feared another pregnancy: "If I can't [keep him away from me] I get pregnant and can't work anymore. If that [happens], who will go to the *milpa?* I have a lot of work and with another child I can't [manage]."

Her home is a small, one-room house with a metal roof and mud walls and floors. The inside is partly divided into kitchen and living areas. A large pile of wood sits to one side of the kitchen; she collects it daily from around the trees surrounding the village, the number of which is rapidly dwindling. During one visit to her home, I took her a dozen eggs, thinking her children could use the protein. On one side of the kitchen was a small wooden table with some plastic containers and the remains of a meal. The living area had a pile of *petates* hastily piled in one corner; cardboard boxes filled with clothes lined the walls.[5] There was a small television on a rough wooden stand near the door; small plastic and beribboned decorations sat next to it. Gloria crouched in front of a square concrete stove—an *estufa*—that she received from a campaigning local politician a few months before. It smoked constantly. The room was stuffy from the smoke, and increasingly hot in the rapidly warming day. She chatted and chatted, while her three youngest daughters skipped around the house. She gleefully told me how, because of the eggs, her *chamacos* could finally eat something other than *enchiladas* (folded tortilla with chili sauce on them)—which they always complained about.[6]

Preparing their children for adulthood is also important for the mothers of Amatlán. Juana struggled with Camila's flightiness during her mid-teenage years—Camila dreamed of marrying for love or of moving to the city to work. Juana said exasperatedly,

> I teach her how to make tortillas because she has to know how to make them because one never knows what her mother-in-law will be like or if her husband will scold her. . . . That is why now I always tell her not to be with the young men because she is too young. It is better to finish one's studies. . . . I don't want her to be with the young men and then to marry too young. . . . Now if she wants to she can sleep or rest but if she gets married she has to cook, go for wood, wash, carry water, and she would never rest. One is always working.

Juana would rather have seen Camila marry after the age of twenty or even twenty-five, stating that young men "only cheat girls and then they disappear." She was especially concerned about Camila's honor and the possibility that she could become pregnant and later be abandoned with no recourse. Camila was an extremely striking teenager and at the age of fourteen was already attracting her fair share of suitors, who Juana would shoo away in frustration, chiding Camila that she was still a *chamaca*—a kid. Eager to get out from under her mother's thumb, Camila made plans to go to work in Mexico City (which she did one summer, as a janitor at the National Polytechnic Institute) or to follow one of her cousins to the United States, where she dreamed of going by airplane. Camila's answer to Juana's entreaties to be sensible was, "If I like [the city] then I'll stay," to which Juana would retort, "In that case, she should not even see it!" The tussle between mother and daughter stemmed from the fact that Camila felt she had choices, while Juana knew that her actual choices were very few and that a woman made choices based on what was available and on one's parents' wishes. And while eventually Camila did marry and have a child at the age of eighteen, she completed high school as Juana wished for her.

In Amatlán, many mothers suffer alongside, or because of, their children. While *marianismo*—the all-suffering, passive motherhood epitomized in the Virgin Mary—is very present in many corners of Latin America, it is not much in evidence in this region. The mothers who do struggle with their children neither view themselves as martyrs nor do they suffer in silence. Esperanza often despaired at the laziness of her son Adrian, one day exclaiming,

"He is no use to me here. He should go away to work but he doesn't want to. I don't know what to do with him." I suggested, "You should stop feeding him." She replied, laughing, "That's true, then he'll go away. . . . [If he is here] I worry when he doesn't get back [or] whether he has been beaten or something. But when he is far away I don't worry. My head can rest."

All the mothers I spoke with worried about their children's future. Emma said, regarding one of her sons who was attending university in the city of Morelia, "A student is a lot of money. My son always asks me for money, 70 pesos, or 50, and it is a lot of money. As he doesn't work. . . . And when there is money we can [help] but often there is none. I tell [my husband] to go to Mexico and to work in a house, or as a bricklayer, to make some money." She added with a smile, "But he says he is too old."

Women in Amatlán were the primary caregivers to children, whether their own or their extended kin; their main duties were domestic. Emma's eldest daughter, Cristina, irritably pointed out that mothers, and women, had to do everything with never any rest. She constantly worried about her children and hoped that they would be able to make something of their lives. But her anxiety was exhausting, as she said, extending her emotion to all aspects of motherhood:

> It's just that as women we have to do everything, get pregnant and be nauseated for the first few months and when everything makes you feel sick. And [cleaning] the pigsty made me feel so sick. And then in the last [months] it is difficult to stand up and do everything. It is so much trouble. And then the pain of the birth, and to breastfeed, and to get up to change the baby in the middle of the night. Your husband is happily asleep but not you. And then to have to control yourself so you don't get pregnant. We [women] have to do everything. There is only the condom and the vasectomy for men, but they don't want them. We have to do it if we don't want to get pregnant. And well, one has to satisfy the husband and also not have so many children.

This centrality of women as caregivers and men as providers is echoed in the structure of Oportunidades. When some of the men of the village on occasion asked to receive the money alongside the women, they were scolded by the authorities and told that it was only for the women. They were told that they should work, not be lazy, and support their families. This response somehow implied that women's natural job at the home could be rewarded and encouraged with money, but men needed to be out in the public sphere without complaint.

The Incompetent Mother: A Look at Dulce's Life

Dulce perfectly illustrates the local constructions of motherhood in this village. She is someone who falls outside the norm of good motherhood—not only by the state's definition but also by the local one. Embodying the notion of problematic motherhood, Dulce's mothering abilities frequently become the topic of conversation. As I mentioned earlier, she is developmentally challenged in some way. It is difficult to know what precisely ails her. People talk about her being *trastornada*—which means disturbed and affected in some behavioral way that makes her different from the norm. She is practically a recluse and refuses to interact with most people, preferring to stay in the safety of her home or that of her parents-in-law—a wonderful elderly couple who speak barely any Spanish. Modesto, Dulce's father-in-law, is a storyteller whose eyes crinkle and shine with impish good humor when he tells a particularly funny or bawdy story.

I was unable to interact with Dulce for more than a few seconds at a time, and during those moments the interaction was mostly at the urging of her husband, a jovial young man who enjoys talking about political issues. Her lack of social skills is evident from her body language. She carries herself in a very meek manner, with hunched shoulders and head down. She never raises her head to look at anyone but rather always looks at the ground. She keeps her long, dark hair in an untidy ponytail low on her neck and wears the same skirt and blouse combination on a daily basis. She is originally from the neighboring village of Zirandaro, which is often used by the people of Amatlán to explain why she is not "normal." Her quirks and misbehaviors can thus easily be chalked up to her being an outsider, someone who is the other.

The villagers' attitude toward her is indulgent and concerned, tinged with criticism for being different. As Mónica said with great disgust on her face, "There are women who have [children] all the time, like the woman over there [Dulce] who does not even look after them or bathe them. The children even have lice." Dulce's sister-in-law Gloria echoed what most other women say about her: how she never bathes her children; that they defecate and urinate inside the house, which she never cleans; and how all the bedding is black with grime. She added, as she shook her head pityingly, "I feel sorry for her, poor thing. She is *trastornada* and used to get fits as a girl. That is why she is this way now." Most criticisms of Dulce revolved around her mothering and how it falls outside of the acceptable and good mothering of the rest of the women of the village.

The medical staff's opinion about Dulce is quite different from those of the villagers. While the people of Amatlán primarily treat her as a helpless, slightly retarded woman who cannot truly help what she does, at the clinic she is seen as someone who is quite savvy and wily. Khiara Bridges (2007), in her research at a New York public hospital, was faced by the folklore surrounding what she refers to as the wily patient—a person seeking health care "whose crushing stupidity is matched only by her formidable duplicity" (4). Patients were classified as stupid by the ancillary staff yet were simultaneously perceived to be "fantastically shrewd manipulators" of the system (6). The patients in Bridges's research were seen to behave in very confusing ways, such as not following orders or not responding as expected, while also being seen as people who, despite their stupidity—and possibly because of it—were artful con artists who would attempt to steal more time and services than was allotted them. Dulce fits perfectly within Bridges's definition: she is *trastornada* but still able to receive medical care and attention for her many children. An early morning exchange between Dulce and the clinic nurse in June 2007 illustrates this image.

As the Tepatepec clinic is about a forty minutes' walk from Amatlán, most people try to get a ride from any of the pickup trucks traveling along the road. That morning, I rushed off after breakfast to catch the first truck to Tepatepec. During the ride, I saw Dulce walking along the road. She was carrying a baby in swaddling clothes while her young son trudged along beside her. Usually, when a truck passes someone walking along the road, the person moves to the side of the road and turns to face the oncoming vehicle to indicate that they would like a ride. But, even though the truck slowed down, Dulce never once looked up nor indicated that she even noticed it.

It took Dulce twenty or thirty minutes more to arrive at the clinic, by which time there were over twelve women waiting to be attended, and the clinic was very busy. On this day, only Nurse Juliana was in attendance, so the young pharmacy attendant/orderly played the role of receptionist/nurse, keeping track of who was next in line and who should be attended to and in what order. When Dulce arrived, she walked up to Juliana and, with her eyes downcast and closely holding her swaddled baby, mumbled that she wanted to go first because "my child has not gone to the bathroom yesterday. I don't know what to do." The following brief exchange took place between them:

Nurse: "Since when has he not gone?"
Dulce: "He didn't go yesterday."

Nurse: "And the day before yesterday he went?"

Dulce: "It seems so."

Nurse (with a slight touch of impatience): "It seems so or he did?"

Not answering the question, Dulce then turned to the woman standing next to her and said, "He is only little; I don't know what I will do."
She looked worried and lost. Her little boy standing next to her was wearing very oversize boots; they looked like they had been inherited from an
older sibling and were his only shoe choice. He looked about four years
old. The baby was lying asleep in Dulce's arms; it was very wrapped up
in a knitted cap on and a blanket. The day was quite warm. After the
above exchange, Nurse Juliana proceeded to ignore Dulce and continued
attending to the patients in their order of arrival. She also did paperwork
for a while.

Once all the other patients were attended to, only Dulce and her little
family remained. They had been sitting for over two hours in the chairs,
watching the proceedings slightly forlornly. During this time no one had
rushed to check her baby or to move Dulce ahead of other patients. The order of arrival at the clinic was strictly kept. No patient took precedence over
another, especially one who was known to be a savvy abuser of the system.

Nurse Juliana eventually turned to Dulce and said, "Let's see, Dulce,
let me see your son, if not you take him to the hospital." Juliana showed
Dulce into the back room where the examining table is. The baby was
crying. Dulce had just been nursing him, and she unlatched him when
she entered through the door. They spent a few minutes inside, while
the nurse checked the baby. As Juliana determined that there was nothing much the matter with the baby, she sent Dulce home. Dulce left
in her usual noiseless manner. Within seconds she was simply a small
figure walking along the road back to Amatlán, her little boy keeping
up with her in his too-large boots.

Juliana sat back down at her nurse's table and, turning to me, disclosed
that Dulce's baby was fine. She said he had normal bowel movements but that

he has a lot of air in his stomach. It is just that she does not get it out.
I showed her how and I told her that after feeding him she should
put him [on her shoulder] and to pat him until he burps. But the
[women here] do it wrong; they do it like this [taps the table with
the flat tips of her fingers] and that is just too gentle. They have to
do it stronger and with a cupped hand to get all the air out. The boy
has colic.

She added, "His testicles are enlarged, and if they do not descend he'll have to be taken to Llano; it can be a hernia." When I commented about Dulce's withdrawn behavior, Juliana scoffed,

> But Dulce *is* intelligent; she *does* understand what one tells her. But her problem is hygiene. I have seen how she lives. She does not drink boiled water; she does not clean [her home]. Other women might live in their small thatch and mud homes but they do care greatly about [their home's] cleanliness. But Dulce's husband can't say anything because when he says something she picks up and goes to her village. She leaves him. So the husband cannot do anything.

In Juliana's eyes, Dulce was not as *trastornada* or retarded as others thought. She saw Dulce as someone much savvier, much more wily than the poor, slow, bad mother seen by others. Reminiscent of the "obtuse, backwards, and altogether unintelligent" female, low-income patients in Bridges's (2007) work in the New York hospital, Dulce is likewise perceived by the nurse as someone who has the ability to manipulate and exploit the system to suit her purposes. She can leave her husband and go back home. The clinicians perceived her to be someone who knows what she wants and will be stubborn enough to get it. This is especially the case with the way she is seen to use her reproductive abilities to her advantage. As with the hyperbolic images of welfare queens—who despite their lack of intelligence still manage to dupe the benevolent government of millions to support their extravagant lifestyles (Bridges 2007)—Dulce's reputation is as someone whose lack of intelligence compels her to shrewdly capitalize on her reproductive capacity to produce children, for which the government, through Oportunidades, generously compensates her.

Dulce's reproduction seemed to be offensive to several women in Amatlán, as evidenced by Ofelia's comments. One day as we discussed family and motherhood, Ofelia said, "That woman does not look after her children, she does not know how to look after them. The children always go about completely filthy (*bien mugrosos*). She is *trastornada* or something. She has that son who can't speak properly, and now she has a little one.[7] She has too many." This statement is highly gendered as it is shaped by assumptions about motherhood and responsibility, as well as the appropriate behaviors for women (Wetterberg 2004). Ofelia's statement has an implied comparison between herself—she prides herself on being a very good mother, one who has been involved in her children's lives from the start—and Dulce—who is decried as not following the necessary tenets for

good motherhood. Even the fact that Dulce is most likely mentally incapable of being fully present in her children's lives and is perhaps unaware
of the dirt that surrounds her life does not exonerate her from criticisms
of poor motherhood. In most people's eyes, she is very far from being the
ever-bountiful, ever-giving, self-sacrificing mother (Bassin et al. 1994) and
instead is an irresponsible fecund dimwit who has too many children. Yet
as Annette Appell (1998) points out, the women classified as "bad" mothers
have become so because they have made bad choices; or because of their
poverty or other factors, they do not have real choices. Thus Dulce's "bad"
mothering can be understood as resulting from her *trastornada* nature,
which prevents her from having any control over her own life, never mind
that of her children.

During the time I was in the field, and even to this day, I was unable to
truly determine what version of Dulce is the real one: the shy and retiring
woman, the hopeless basket case, or the wily abuser of the system. It seemed
that everyone had their own opinion of her, though the one thing everyone
agreed on was that her mothering left much to be desired. Her wiliness almost becomes that of the trickster figure—the one who is halfway between
two polar opposites and thus must "retain some of that duality, namely an
ambiguous and equivocal character" (Levi-Strauss 1955:441). Her ambiguity
is even greater, as she follows the rules of compliance set up by Oportunidades but is not obedient in the larger sense, that is, she is often pregnant and
is constantly producing children. She thus (unconsciously) toes the line and
receives money from the government. By slipping through these gaps, Dulce
can get what she wants, despite the consequences; because of her undesirable
mothering, she can get the Mexican state to help through Oportunidades.
Hence, despite being considered a bad mother, she still qualifies for receiving the stipends and thus provides for her children—at least officially. These
contradictions make her especially interesting.

Moving Out of a Cardboard House: Frida's Story

Frida is a curious example of the connection between motherhood
and the larger system. Her story is a sad one. Her husband, Casimiro, is
regularly drunk and abusive, beating her, and her children, frequently.
A somewhat bombastic, big-talking man who does not own farmland,
he makes a meager living from itinerant work on other people's *milpas*.
People whispered that he had once strangled a woman to death, and thus
many feared his violence. Esperanza said, "[Casimiro] is very aggressive.

If you go to his house . . . to collect your debts they say he chases you with a machete. He does not want to pay his debts. That is why when Frida receives her Oportunidades, you can see how everyone runs after her to be paid back. But even with that she does not pay them. She does not let go of her money!" To make ends meet, and to supplement her money from Oportunidades, Frida makes bread and washes others' clothes. This means that she is out of the house, working, and does not always have time to do housework. Consequently, her husband often comes home to no tortillas, fueling his anger and provoking violent outbursts. She is a slight woman in her mid-thirties, who dresses in knee-length straight skirts and tank tops. She always has her hair tightly pulled back and gelled into a ponytail. While she smiles readily, there is always a slight impression of desperation and hunger in her smile. It is not a happy smile.

Her house is one of the most impoverished of the village. While most homes are located in the grid that makes up the village—and are on plots of equal rectangular size to their neighbors—Frida's house is on the very edge of the village. It sits on a small bluff overlooking the river and is surrounded by a lot of scrubby, denuded land. She is neighbor to Dulce, whose house is indeed at the edge of town. Despite the fact that this is a tiny village, this is still considered to be the "boondocks" and the least desirable part to live in. The home consists of two small huts—the living quarters and the kitchen—made of bamboo logs woven together. Nowadays, most homes in the village are made of concrete, or if they are older houses, they are made of very sturdy wattle and daub with thatch roofs. This particular set of houses was very rickety and completely exposed to the elements. It was dismissively described as a cardboard house by Caridad, one of my *comadres* and Frida's neighbor across the street. While the living area was built on a slight platform made of dried mud, it did not seem high enough off the ground to prevent water from running through it during the torrential summer rains this area experiences.

Frida was always very inviting when I visited. She would set out all her plastic chairs and offer bread and coffee—which she could ill afford. The living quarters were practically devoid of material possessions. There was no TV or any accouterments of modern life. The mud floor simply housed a few rolled up *petlatl* and, rather surprisingly, a very well set up camp bed covered in thick blankets in one corner. When I admired it during one visit, Frida proudly said that it belonged to her eldest daughter and had been given to her by her *madrina*, the wife of the primary teacher Maestro Bernabé. The teacher's wife, concerned about the sleeping arrangements of the family, insisted on giving the girl the bed so she would not become ill and would grow healthily. It was one of Frida's most prized possessions.

Frida is not originally from Amatlán but began living there after marrying Casimiro under unusual circumstances. She said that she is from Papalotl, about a three hours' walk away. She said that when she was sixteen, she

> used to go to Llano to sell *pilón*, since my father ground [sugar cane].[8] And my husband went because he would go with [Gastón] who sells things [in the markets]. And he would come to see me in the market. And one day he gave me some soda, but I told him I did not know him and I [asked him] why he gave me soda. And, well, he tricked me, and that is why I am here.

Casimiro is eleven years her senior, so when they met he was twenty-seven. She later explained what his trickery had consisted of. She said,

> He told me that his sisters-in-law were sick and [asked] whether I wanted to come to help. My mother did not want me to come, and neither did I. But I came and I stayed with some aunts. And I helped [Casimiro's family] for about four days. But then they did not let me leave. And my mother came and then she said that I couldn't leave any more, that I was here to stay. And [Casimiro] locked me up. And like that I stayed [here]. I never returned to Papalotl.

From Frida's story, there is a sense that her honor was compromised by going to a man's house—even in as innocent a manner as the one she described. Thus she would no longer be a good woman and would not be able to return home. Wedding ceremonies are not very common in Amatlán, with the majority of marriages being common-law. Sandstrom (1991) noted that couples would begin to live together in the house of the groom's parents or would elope to a new house and would subsequently be considered by the community to be married. Frida possibly fell between the cracks of this classification, as living in close proximity to Casimiro and his family would have implied an acquiescence to couplehood, and because she was in a village not her own, it might have been seen as a form of elopement. She maintained, however, that she was not a willing participant in the transaction.

Frida's status as a possession of Casimiro has continued to this day. When I asked her how many children she considered to be the ideal number, she said,

More than four. My husband only wants four. He took me to be sterilized. I did not want to go, but he forced me to go. I was scared and I did not want to; but he wanted it and he took me to Chicón. It was not a very large [cut]; they only open you up a little bit. But I can no longer have any children. If they had not operated on me I might already have about three more. This was about eight years ago. . . . I wanted many [children]. But one of my daughters died. She was only seven months old and she began to vomit, who knows why. And not even with the doctor did she get better. And [her fontanelle] sunk in and it looked like a little bowl. And here where we swallow (the throat) was also sunk in. And she died. She would be fifteen now.

This girl, whose name Frida never shared with me, was her second child. She now has four children: three girls and one boy.

Frida considers herself a very good mother. Despite being one of the poorest women in Amatlán, she uses any means she has at her disposal to make ends meet and gain some small amount of status in the process. She constantly searches for income-generating projects, joining with other women to make products to earn money. Her primary means of gaining status, however, is through patronage. This patronage takes two forms: *compadrazgo* (godparenthood) and political clientelism.

If there is a women's project to earn money, Frida is likely to be part of the group. During the time I knew her in Amatlán, she joined any money-making opportunity she could find. Two projects were slightly more successful than others: making bread and sewing. In 2005, a group of women got together through some outside funding to fix up the bakery—which is next door to the *Casa de Salud*—to make and sell bread. They would pool their money to buy the ingredients, and every three days they would spend most of the day kneading, forming, and selling the bread—small, sweet or savory pieces that melted in the mouth. I found it impossible to eat only one. During the following two days, they would walk around the village selling bread to people in Amatlán. They would take turns carrying large, heavy baskets of very hot bread on their backs to sell to people in neighboring villages. And while the women worked very hard at this backbreaking job, with the money they made selling the bread, they barely broke even. When I asked the seven participating women, which included Lourdes, Frida, and Marcelina (the *auxiliar*), why they engaged in such tiring work for so little reward, they good-humoredly answered that it was fun and it kept them busy. But the project did not last long. The funding dried up, and the women began to fight with each other about money gone missing.

Frida told me, "I was happy making bread. And any money made was put into a box. And three of the women had access to the box. And when there was enough accumulation of pesos and we wanted to divide it, they only gave some of us 700 pesos. They gave others more. And that is why we did not want this anymore; we had a fight." This eventually built up a general mistrust, bringing about the demise of the bakery project.

Frida also was an active part of the sewing group that emerged in early 2007. This sewing cooperative had been established by a teacher from Xalapa—the state capital. Its purpose was to be an egalitarian group where everyone would reap rewards equally—though the cloth, thread, and designs were all provided by the teacher, who was also the middleman between the women and the eventual buyers. About twenty women had joined and spent every afternoon embroidering napkins and tablecloths. Yet by the end of the summer, the group had dwindled to only a handful of women. Most women blamed Fabiola, a particularly strong-willed woman, for the exodus. She managed to gain the ear of the Xalapa teacher and so became that person's voice and representative and, in effect, the leader of the group. All egalitarianism was lost. The women accused her of being too difficult and of taking over and wanting all the money for herself.

Frida has always been an energetic embroiderer, selling cloths to anyone who will buy them. When I visited her at home, she would often be sitting on a small chair, sewing the edges onto a cloth, while showing her daughters how to do the same. Frida and Fabiola used to be very good friends before the sewing group. But Frida was particularly critical of the way Fabiola had managed the group. She said she had joined because it was potentially good income. She added that she was one of twenty-seven other women who joined. But that number had eventually decreased to eleven because Fabiola insisted that there was not enough money for all of them; she forced several women out, while others—including Frida—dropped out over time of their own accord. This made Frida particularly bitter, as she needs the income to help her feed and clothe her children.

What sets Frida apart from the other women in the community is her practically palpable desperation to make money. Most of the women seem comfortable with their lack of money, using humor to poke fun at their poverty and lack of buying power. Frida has a hunger for money and for physical possessions that tends to bother the other women. She primarily survives through a series of tactics—these are short-term expedient methods (begging, borrowing, and so on) to manage her day-to-day life. She has very little scope in her life for strategies, which require long-term planning and which tend to require greater agentive power (see Nancy Scheper-Hughes 1993 for her distinction between tactics and strategies used by marginalized women in a Brazilian slum). Frida is one of the few people in the community who is not embarrassed to borrow money from others. Begging and borrowing are not shameful when one cannot afford shame. Her primary method of enticing lenders is to use her children as hooks to pull at people's heartstrings and bend them toward generosity. She will dress the children in their tattiest clothes and then have them ask for money or other things (fruit or corn, for example), always with the promise to pay it back. But she has a reputation for never repaying, so her lenders are few and far between. I found myself lending her money and giving her copies of photos I had taken of her children on many occasions, despite Esperanza's repeated comments that I would never see the money again. While I never was repaid monetarily, I participated in several events that Frida organized and was repaid through the reciprocal circulation of favors and food.

Frida's desperate need for money and status results in her using the system to her advantage. Here is where her incipient efforts at strategic thinking arise. These efforts are only mildly successful, yet she expends great energy in them. She has always been very politically active, yet this participation is solely to achieve personal gains, not because of any particular interest in politics. This is different from Fabiola, who, while also participating in politics for the monetary and material gains, is interested in politicking for its own sake. Frida is out only to gain as much as she can. Because politics in Mexico have historically functioned through political clientelism (Schedler 2004), politicians often promise and give out material benefits to anyone who promises to vote for them. Frida did not care for strict political affiliation, and so over the years I knew her in Amatlán, she switched from the PRI to the PAN on various occasions. In 2007, she was an ardent follower of the PAN candidate. He had promised his voters to give them a *vivienda*—a house, which meant money to buy materials to build a concrete house. This appealed to Frida as she could upgrade from her "*casa de cartón*"—the cardboard house of Caridad's uncharitable words.

In the past, Fabiola and Frida were best of friends because they were both *PRI-istas*—they voted for the PRI. But with Frida's transition to the PAN (or any other party that will help her), they are enemies. Each of them became a village spokesman for her party, enticing women to vote for particular candidates. Frida knew that if she had a leadership position, she would gain even more political favor and possibly have more money to build her house and fill it with goods. It was not unusual to see her visiting women and telling them to vote for the PAN. She often used the (empty) threat of taking away their Oportunidades if they did not vote accordingly. She was always very proud of being able to milk the politicians for what they were worth. Yet other women saw her forays into politics as futile. Caridad simply laughed at politics and preferred not to get involved. She said that it seemed a waste of time to keep on following politicians because usually one would have nothing to show for it. One only had to look at Frida to see that despite always supporting candidates, she still lived in a *casa de cartón*.

The system of *compadrazgo*—godparenthood—was especially useful for Frida to gain goods for her children and status for her family. She searches for *padrinos* with high social and economic capital so they can help her get ahead. *Compadrazgo* is also a much safer bet than politics, as *compadres* are much more honor bound than politicians to fulfill their promises. She is very opportunistic in asking people to be godparents for her children. While the concept of a godparent originally had religious roots, it has been co-opted by the Mexican school system and has become a remarkably popular secular institution. Whenever children graduate from school— whether from kindergarten or high school—they need a *padrino* to walk across the graduation stage with them to receive their diplomas. The role of the *padrino* is to subsequently give occasional gifts, money, and other forms of support to their godchild over the years. While some people simply ask a close relative or friend to serve as the godparent, not expecting much from the person except for him or her to serve in the graduation, others are more strategic in choosing people with social and economic capital. There were a few people who were always in demand for the role, and Maestro Bernabé, the head teacher at the primary school in Amatlán, was one of them, sometimes serving as godfather to children graduating from every stage in one year. Frida had been asking him for years to be godfather to her eldest daughter, Gracia. She knew that he would take the role very seriously, as evidenced by the bed he and his wife bought her.

In Frida's eyes, the *padrinos* are vital to help her children get ahead in life. They are "ritual sponsors," who cement relationships and "build social bridges" (Kemper 1982:18, 21) between kin not related by blood. They can provide money, material goods, and status—which helps the family build networks that open doors for future endeavors. From my conversations with Frida, I gathered that she was not necessarily thinking long-term for her children's future, perhaps because her children are still young. Her main concerns tended to revolve around tangible things, such as money or goods. Frida's good motherhood is evident through her constant concern for her children's welfare.

Both Frida and Dulce's mothering are problematic to the neat dichotomous categories of "good" and "bad" mothers; indeed, Dulce is possibly an example of a bad mother by local standards, within a larger category of (indigenous) bad mothers. However, Frida and Dulce are not average Amatlán mothers: both are literally and socially marginal (they are not from Amatlán, their houses are on the edge of town, and they are the poorest of the poor). They are marginal mothers. By their exceptional status they bring into focus local and national concerns about motherhood and modernity. And perhaps, also, they make other mothers in Amatlán look good by comparison. Though much of the strength of redefining motherhood has been on the state level, within Dulce and Frida's lives exist the complications about the sites of control and surveillance and how community members themselves also engage in the defining process. Dulce's story and the ways the other women judge her a "bad mother" shows the complications embedded within definitions of motherhood. Frida's story is equally compelling as it sheds light on the challenges of being a "good mother" when faced with domestic violence and alcoholism.

Helping to Keep Baby Healthy and Clean: Molding Good Mothers

Indigenous forms of mothering the world over have been challenged and sometimes transformed "in the name of civilization, modernity, and scientific medicine" (Jolly 1998:1). Society creates concepts such as good and bad mothers; these concepts shape the ways that certain women—especially those from marginalized backgrounds who strive to be part of the mainstream—behave. Society is particularly strict on mothers, holding them up to high—and, oftentimes, nearly impossible—standards. For example, Japanese mothers are involved in the country's education system and are simultaneously shaped into good mothers through their extremely regimented involvement in their children's home and school lives. During this process, women "act as culturally constructed mothers and self-sacrificing managers of home, family, and children" (Allison 1996:7). Sudanese women in Boddy's account (2007:179) exist at the crossroads of British colonial efforts to "civilize" the country and the "fatal obstacle" of the practice of female genital cutting. Boddy shows how a woman's mind was seen to be "ruled by her breeding parts," and thus her domestic space had to be normalized before she could produce normal and rational children. In Mexico, Oportunidades promotes "normative assumptions concerning 'women's roles' so that the work women undertake, in ensuring that children's needs are met, is taken for granted as something that mothers 'do'" (Molyneux 2006:438). The problem with these assumptions is that the social relations of reproduction remain unproblematized, and women's work is simply naturalized.

In Japan, the state became particularly concerned with the role of mothers in the modernization of the country. The origins of the state's involvement in Japanese mothers' lives is *ryosai kenbo*, or "good wives, wise mothers," which was a government-sponsored ideology during the Meiji period (1868–1912) as the country was modernizing. As Deborah Shamoon, a scholar of modern Japanese gender and culture, stated, its purpose was to promote education and hygiene for women to make them better mothers, better able to raise strong soldiers for the nation (Deborah Shamoon, personal communication, October 13, 2010). They were meant to be the "epitome of virtuous womanhood" (Ivry 2007:254). While *ryosai kenbo* allowed women to exercise authority in their own home and over their own children—a vast improvement over their previous status as little more than a "borrowed womb"—this ideology denied women any legal standing, placing them in the same category as the deformed or mentally incompetent. The power rested in the hands of the male head of the household (Lock 1990:44). This ideology was reincarnated in the 1970s with the concept of the "professional housewife [*sengyô shuhu*]" whose work is solely in the home and whose energy is completely geared to her husband's career and children's education (Ivry 2007:254). Even in contemporary Japan, where increasing numbers of women enter the workforce, the pressure remains for them to be good mothers despite their employment outside the home (Fujita 1989).

The roots of this ideology of motherhood lie in standardization and social control (Lock 1990), and the emphasis is on stability of the social and family structure, much like the Healthy Marriage Initiative in the United States. This initiative, begun in the mid-1990s, encouraged people from lower-income backgrounds to marry, because "marriage is an essential institution of a successful society which promotes the interests of children" (Administration for Children and Families 2012). Former U.S. president George W. Bush, a strong proponent of the initiative, stated in a proclamation, "Many one-parent families are also a source of comfort and reassurance, yet a family with a mom and dad who are committed to marriage and devote themselves to their children helps provide children a sound foundation for success" (White House 2001). The initiative's arguments are similar to those of many development programs, where the responsibility for the production of good citizens is placed at women's doors. Mothers around the world are seen as everything to everyone: they hold the family together; they work hard; they feed and clothe their children; they protect their children and give them shelter while also allowing them to grow and flourish. But any misstep, and they become "dangerous": they overprotect, they shield, they build metaphorical walls, and instead of helping to give their children wings, they cut them so they are stunted—and thus the children grow to become stunted adults. It is easy to blame mothers. They walk such a tight balance and are so scrutinized by society that any lapse can result in anything from social stigma to ostracism and even to legal consequences.

The idea of bad mothering has been explored by a variety of anthropologists, including Nancy Scheper-Hughes (1993), Anna Tsing (1990), Cecilia Van Hollen (2003), and Christa Craven (2005). Feminist sociologists and historians have also analyzed this concept, particularly looking at welfare mothers, lesbian mothers, and working mothers (see Ladd-Taylor and Umansky 1998). A "bad mother" is someone who fails at carrying out expected social roles; this failure is frequently perceived to be caused by her selfish and uncaring attitude toward her children and society at large—what Chavez (2004) refers to as pathological reproductive behavior. These cases where certain women are classified as bad mothers allow us to understand the various ways mainstream norms are used as the standards for behavior for all women—especially those who are seen to clearly fall outside of the acceptable norm.

Anna Tsing (1990:283) analyzed the concept of bad motherhood among American women charged with endangering their newborns by having unassisted births. The "monster stories" emerging from these situations were quickly taken up by the media and general public, whereby discourses of fetus and child protection overlapped with the medical model of a supervised birth process. It is at this juncture between the media, medicine, and the law that the image of a "vulnerable infant, endangered by its maternal environment unless rescued by altruistic outsiders" has emerged. In a similar manner, indigenous and low-income women in Mexico are constantly reminded that their actions carry risk, and so they must modify them for the betterment of their children and society. As Linda Whiteford (1996:250) points out in her political and economic analysis of a Florida law for drug-addicted pregnant women, this classification of women as bad mothers simply creates a scapegoat instead of focusing society's attention on the "effects of racism, classism, and sexism" on some of the most vulnerable members of our society.

A sharp dichotomy exists between good and bad mothers. Rebecca Kukla, in her book *Mass Hysteria* (2005), illustrates this dichotomy by discussing what she calls "the fetish mother" and the "unruly mother." The fetish mother is the natural mother, who bonds naturally with her child, and her body symbolizes the "well-ordered human nature free from hysterical incoherence . . . or deformed monstrosity (82)." This mythified and idealized mother gains fulfillment and satisfaction in caring for her children (Bassin et al. 1994) and in a paradoxical sense almost seems to become better and stronger the more she sacrifices for them; her "suffering is not a negation but an affirmation . . . [and] by connecting the earthly and the sacred, the mother's power becomes visible" (Nadal-Melsió 1996:88). The unruly mother is capricious and difficult and must be "carefully regulated, policed, and controlled" so her hysteria cannot affect her offspring and the body politic (Kukla 2005:83). This image of problematic motherhood is represented by the welfare queens, the unstable parturients, or the drug-addled women of society. Though contrasting, both images are fictions.

It is precisely this concept of child vulnerability that is espoused by the Mexican discourses of development. Though there is no denying that Mexico has extremely marginalized and disadvantaged populations whose children are particularly susceptible to illness and malnutrition, these discourses tend to ignore larger historical or structural processes that have caused these marginalities and instead place their focus on the mothers' abilities, or perceived lack thereof. These women are seen as unruly mothers in need of perpetual supervision by the state apparatus. With the help of the *pláticas* and behavioral changes expected in exchange for the cash, enrolled mothers can be resocialized and reshaped into compliant, obedient women and mothers.

The Mexican government's view about the women enrolled in Oportunidades is very similar to the views held in the United States about welfare mothers and those whose children have been taken by the child welfare system. As Appell (1998) illustrates in her research on mothers receiving welfare, these women's parenting is more visible to the government than that of their middle-class counterparts because their lives intersect with government agencies on a regular basis. Within this framework, if it is the mothers who are the problem, then it is *they* who must be fixed. But to be fixed they must become different women, and thus failure is "usually a foregone conclusion" (Appell 1998:376). When women are told that they have failed, they often respond by intensifying their efforts to achieve this perfection; but if this perfection is not reached, it creates a destructive cycle of mothers being blamed by others and by themselves. (Bassin et al. 1994:3).

Within the Mexican imagination, mothers are revered, often held up as paragons of virtue; they are the embodiment of the Virgin Mary—chaste, pure, devoted, and self-sacrificing. Such images of motherhood seem to be especially present among middle- and upper-class women, who can usually afford to be in agreement with these impossible myths—they have money, servants, and time.[9] While the Mexican working class or rural poor people also consider mothers to be important, they are not held up to impossible standards. As Collins (1994) shows, their motherhood cannot be analyzed in isolation from their social, political, and economic contexts. Their "motherhood occurs in specific historical contexts framed by interlocking structures of race, class, and gender" (56). The Amatlán women's lived experiences and their grounded realities include hands scrubbed raw from washing clothes and burned from making tortillas. For them, work and family are not separate spheres but are instead intertwined and, indeed, form part of what Collins (1994:59) refers to as "motherwork"—the ways that women work to maintain family life against forces that might undermine its integrity. With feet firmly planted in the earth of their *solares*, these women certainly do not have time to reflect on the ideal motherhood.

Oportunidades's goal is to encourage the "government of the family," which Foucault terms *economy* (1991:92) and defines as the correct manner of managing individuals, wealth, and goods within a family, promoting the good management of the state. Foucault argues that the art of governing flows upward and downward: to govern a state, a person must know how to govern oneself. The mothers of Oportunidades are expected to follow the good example of the state and prepare good citizens for its future. This scalar system—from state to family and individual level—has within it embedded structures of surveillance and control, which are, in Foucault's words, "as attentive as that of the head of a family over his household and his goods" (1991:92).

If Foucault outlines the broader structures that supervise, discipline, and punish people, it is Gramsci's notions of hegemony that speak to matters of compliance more directly. Gramsci speaks of the ways people comply and become subjects even while they seemingly understand their subjectification. The Gramscian notion of hegemony "induces people to comply with a dominant set of practices and institutions without the threat of physical force" (Litowitz 2000:515). This type of hegemony induces passive compliance not through any direct act of force but by taking over various parts of civil society—churches, schools, clubs, and so on—that act in a diffuse way over people's choices. This "spontaneous consent" given by the most dispossessed segments of the population to the directives of the dominant segment is "historically caused" by the prestige that the dominant segment enjoys "because of its position and function in the world of production" (Gramsci 1978:12).

The reproductive habitus model I have proposed allows one to frame how the women's bodily micropractices are shaped by larger forces. All these forces—the class and social structures, gender roles, and government policies—become even more pronounced when the women are part of Oportunidades. Once a woman is enrolled, there are only a few set paths she can take to actually be seen as a good mother. In this system, good mothers do not *need* to be directly disciplined through repressive mechanisms. Rather than operating through violence or seizure of the women's bodies or bodily processes, these disciplinary technologies work by "producing new objects and subjects of knowledge, by inciting and channeling desires, generating and focusing individual and group energies, and establishing bodily norms and techniques for observation, monitoring, and controlling bodily movements, processes, and capacities" (Sawicki 1999:193). Such practices render the body "more useful, more powerful, and more docile" (193).

The Oportunidades program functions very effectively in shaping motherhood by using a carrot (giving mothers money) and a stick (taking away the mothers' money). The system does not return to its original condition even when the stipend is taken away because the money has become part of the system. It is not just an external infusion of cash that the people can take or leave; its regularity ensures that it becomes a large part of the women's family income. Moreover, these systems—whether medical technologies, economic development programs, or medical encounters—secure control of the enrolled populations through the production of new norms of motherhood, by redefining women within their identity as mothers, and by offering "specific kinds of solutions to problems they face" (Sawicki 1999:194). This situation thus creates a powerful incentive for the women to comply and holds within it dire consequences for any perceived noncompliance. It becomes all the more powerful in contexts where women's political subjectification becomes localized at the site of birth: when they literally become the producers of modern citizens. The compliance in the creation of children-citizens is ensured by medicalizing the reproductive corpus during pregnancy and during the act of birth itself.

The many people who act as forces in the women's lives—the physicians, nurses, and teachers—would be some of the first people to state that these women are not good mothers. While in the day-to-day these people would say the women are good enough mothers (with the implication of "partially good or barely sufficient" [Barlow 2004:522])—because the children are generally healthy and well fed—these people would not regard the women as good mothers in a larger sense. They would say that yes, they feed their children, but not the right amount of meats and legumes, or yes, their children are healthy, but they are prone to tuberculosis and coughs because of breathing in the smoke from cooking fires. So the women constantly have to battle the accusation of being barely good enough mothers, or outright bad and problematic mothers, because they are considered too fertile, too ignorant, and too uncultured to realize that they are causing and perpetuating their own poverty. These women are seen as perpetuating their poverty by choice. This idea is epitomized by the physician's words I shared earlier: "It's just that they do not want to develop. They are this way because they want to be. . . . They just stay at home, marginalized, and have kids."[10]

This physician's quote reveals many of the implicit assumptions about mothers in general, and indigenous women in particular. There is an unspoken comparison between the private sphere of women, who as mothers stay at home and multiply the population through their biopotentiality (by "breeding like ants" or "having children like a *tlacuache* [opossum]" as some of the women verbalized), and the public sphere of men, who go to the fields, migrate out of the region, and are free to create culture. And while this gendered division of labor is normative in this region, the physician's words reveal a value judgment about the women's lives. What would the physician suggest they should be doing? "Home" as opposed to what? The word *marginada* (marginalized) is also revealing about how marginalization is used in everyday speech in Mexico. Likely emerging from a similar construct of nationality as *indigenismo* did, it implies that somehow the women choose to be marginal rather than acknowledging that there are forces that make them marginal. Within this notion of mothers as marginalized also exists a binary opposition, where good mothers are advanced, developed, compliant, and modern, and bad mothers are underdeveloped, backward, noncompliant, and unmodern. Such rhetoric victimizes the women and blames them for the larger structure within which they live.

CHAPTER 5

Laughter and the "Best" Medicine

"No one is at the clinic"

ONE DAY IN EARLY 2004, THE VILLAGE WOMEN WERE ASKED TO ATTEND an important gathering at the *Casa de Salud.* The physician and nurse from the Tepatepec clinic were to come up to give check-ups, and the women were expected to attend. When Esperanza and I arrived, there were only about five women waiting outside the *casa.* Some were sitting on a log in the shade, while others stood next to them. They were all chatting quietly. There were a few women inside the *casa* itself—which was open that day. Esperanza and I joined the women in the shade. At first we stood, but since it appeared that all of us would be there for a while, we moved to the roughly hewn wooden benches placed across from the *casa.* We sat there for a long time. Women came and went; some entered the *casa,* while others joined us. The group was never larger than a dozen women. Used to waiting long periods for medical care, the women simply sat and chatted with one another. They talked about what they were doing there and the sorts of health-related behaviors they were expected to follow, as well as about the weather and village gossip. The women somehow seemed to know whose turn it was next, as no one called out to the women from the *casa.* In fact, the *casa* seemed surprisingly devoid of activity. Yet the group of women diminished slowly. Soon only Esperanza and two other women remained. There was a slight impatience setting in with the three women. They joked about how they always spent their time waiting for medical care and how sometimes even after they waited for a long time, they were told to go home and come back another day. This prompted Esperanza—usually a very shy woman who is rarely demanding—to walk across to the *casa* to see what was going on. While she did not manage to gain admittance to the *casa*, she did learn that apparently all the women were supposed to go by the Tepatepec clinic on Saturday for the inauguration of the National Vaccination Week.

Eventually Doctor Braulio, a tall, thin man in his mid-forties, came out and looked at Esperanza's *cartilla* (a government-issued card containing a person's medical history) and those of the two other women there. He went over the *cartillas* perfunctorily and made a few comments about what the women's overall health looked like. After this, all three women sat down on the benches again and chatted, mainly about health and *cartillas*. One of the women was Fabiola.

Fabiola is a woman in her late thirties whose most striking features are her eyes, which can only be described as dewy, deer-caught-in-the-headlights eyes. But her eyes belie the core of steel that runs through this woman. She is known throughout the village as a formidable foe who should not be crossed. She has a reputation for being a controlling and bossy woman. She has had run-ins with most women in the village. The reason given for her strong (even difficult) character—which is considered very unusual and even improper—is that she is not from Amatlán but is instead from the village of Mandarinas, which everyone agrees produces difficult women. She is strong and assertive and is heavily engaged in politics—whether village gossip or state-level government. She rallies behind the political candidates who she feels will give her the most benefits. She determines this measure from the candidates' "donation" of goods—ranging from food baskets and plastic storage containers to "environmental" *estufas* (ovens) made of concrete—to her and other voters. Most women in the village avoid entering into any discussion or project with Fabiola, as they have learned from experience that she always gets her own way. One year, when she tried to become the *promotora*, she did not have support. As one of the women said, "When they asked [us] to raise our hand if we wanted her, no one raised it. They wanted Ofelia to be the *vocal*.[1] Because if not Fabiola would have reported [on] all [the women at the clinic]."

That day at the *casa* gathering, Fabiola began to tell us that she had been given an operation appointment a long time ago to reduce her breast size. Gesturing at her breasts, she said how uncomfortable they were and how much back and hip pain they caused. As she described her discomfort, she smiled and then laughed. She said that she had not had surgery because she could never find anyone at the Tepatepec clinic to give her the paperwork to go to the hospital in Poza Rica. Nodding in agreement, the other women laughed with her. They all knew how many times they had gone to the clinic only to be disappointed.

As Doctor Braulio joined them on the bench, the women discussed how it was very common for them to walk all the way to the clinic and find no physician and no nurse there when they arrived. They laughed in commiseration as they said how much of a wasted day that usually was for them. They seemed to have no problem saying this very critical statement in front of Doctor Braulio. Instead, his presence catalyzed them to list criticisms about the clinic and health care in general. Each time a new point was brought up by one woman, the others would nod and erupt into laughter, spurring them on to add more complaints to their ever-growing list. Fabiola topped the list by telling a story of how it took her forever to convince her husband to go to the clinic for a long-overdue visit, and then when he got there, he found no one to attend to him. She said he returned extremely disgruntled with the clinicians for not working and with her for wasting his day. All the women, including her, laughed when she added that there was no money for anything related to health care anyway—so having no one at the clinic might be a benefit after all. Doctor Braulio interjected to remind her to tell her husband to go on the following Saturday to the clinic to have a check-up. As the clinic is usually closed on Saturdays, the women answered, "But there will be no one there." He replied slightly impatiently, "And when is it that you are meant to go [to the vaccination event]?" The women responded in unison, "On Saturday," to which he said, "Then . . . ?" The women responded to this rebuke by bursting into laughter.[2]

People laughed for many reasons. Sometimes things are just funny, and everyone finds them so: a woman falling off of a chair, for example. Sometimes things are not quite so funny, but people laugh to commiserate or because they have somehow experienced this before: people laugh when they travel for miles to the health centers only to find no one there. They have all experienced this, and they expect this from those who control their lives. They have always been buffeted by the changing fads of the state, and they expect no less from the current fads and programs. And sometimes humor is just a useful way to cope with the vagaries of life: laughing at those in power helps to make one feel better. Instead of viewing humor simply as a way to manage difficulty, agency is contextual for these women—in some contexts they can be agents, while in others their agency is reduced or stripped. Humor therefore exists beyond coping and functions to build a community among the women—as if to say "we have all suffered and so we can all laugh about it together."

Laughter Forming a Bond

The women's words in this book give insight into the constant tussle between women's desires, their compliance, and their perceived disobedience. On the one hand are the various policies that interact to constrict women's choices in such a way that their compliance comes hand-in-hand with coercion. The women find themselves being compliant to policies and practices that they oftentimes do not agree with. On the other hand is the women's perceived disobedience regarding their reproductive lives. The women have been painted as overly reproductive and extremely fertile, as only women from the rural backwoods of Mexico can be. The stratified reproduction within which these women exist shapes the way that they interact with the larger system. Within this system, the women often have very little recourse. They are caught in a situation where they have to comply and follow orders. Few, if any, of the women ever disobey medical orders outright. Disobedience, for them, comes at a price.

In development and public health, laughter, gossip, rumors, and other forms of invisible communication are often seen as signs of ignorance. They are seen as trivial. Anthropologists, however, see these forms of communication as important places to understand the workings of power. Humor exists in the margins and allows one to examine the spaces between expectation and reality. Joel Sherzer (2002:150) notes that humor among the Kuna "is not compartmentalized . . . , restricted to particular specific or marginal occasions and places." Humor is not just "time out and time off from the serious stuff of life" (150) but is instead a way to comment on misfortune and disaster; it is also a means to (possibly) exaggerate and comment on social and cultural realities.

Davies (1990) discusses a close association between ethnic jokes and social stratification. While a subordinate group might accept or reject the legitimacy of the elite classes, they are usually powerless to do much about it. They are therefore confronted by the gap between their own ways of life and those of the powerful. Jokes can often bridge this gap for them. By laughing, the women are able to mock the structures that constrict them, they can find solidarity and community with others, and they can resist— at least in part—some of the difficulties they encounter. Besides its role as a weapon of the weak, by defusing anger and frustration, laughter also lessens discontent. Nonetheless, in doing so, it can foster complacency, which can once again feed back into making the women compliant.

In his 1905 book *The Joke and Its Relation to the Unconscious*, Sigmund Freud makes a very detailed psychological analysis of the use of jokes and witticism. He shows how humor is used effectively in attacking "the great, the dignified, and the mighty" (Freud 2003:100). The joke is thus a rebellion against authority and a way to be liberated from one's oppression. Humor has been actively used as social protest where the marginalized mock the powerful and thus play with the social hierarchy by turning it upside down (Hart 2007)—such as during Carnival, when people can dress up as the oligarchs and jeer at their ways. Humor, though considered a weapon of the weak, is also a much more effective method of removing obstacles than serious criticism is. This is because "criticism expressed in a joking manner is more difficult to refute by 'rational' arguments. Authority and power can melt, as the invitation to laugh with one another appeals to all human feelings and breaks down 'official' barriers" (Hart 2007:8).

Jokes about lived situations and experiences tend to be ambiguous. They do not openly criticize life but rather poke gentle fun at a situation. The women can thus laugh with Fabiola because they share her frustration with the clinic, yet they can do so in front of the physician because they cloak their criticism in laughter. Because of this ambiguity, jokes can act as a respite from social pressures, whether overt or covert (Hart 2007). Laughter also allows the formation of a bond and fellowship, as Konrad Lorenz (1974:293) stated, while simultaneously drawing a line—laughter bonds the women and separates them from the physician, the butt of their jokes.

Laughter and jokes are important vehicles for self-analysis of an individual or a group and are about "complex human 'problem[s]' whose presence in [one's] life is a source of pressing concern" (Basso 1979:17). Keith Basso in his work among the Apache showed that by imitating the Anglo-Americans who come into contact with them—and who view the Apache with a certain amount of disdain or pity—Apache jokers use jokes to make sense of these people. Jokes are simultaneously funny and dangerous, especially when one is poking fun at someone with the ability to hurt. Alan Sandstrom (1991), while researching religious practices and identity in Amatlán in the 1970s and 1980s, points out that the people considered it dangerous to criticize the *mestizos* and the system. His rich ethnography tells of countless instances where to speak out was to be hurt, even murdered, and thus people learned to speak in undercurrents about their *mestizo* neighbors. While he does not discuss the role of humor in these comments, he notes that the people engaged in hyperbolic descriptions of what they considered the dangerous urban centers and their *mestizo* inhabitants. Perhaps over time, with the greater contact that the indigenous population has with the *mestizos*, the people have become more comfortable with using humor to poke fun at the system and its representatives. The jokes and humorous stories they tell are funny, yet if heard by the wrong ears—those of the physicians or representatives of Oportunidades— could potentially become dangerous.

Acting as a barometer, humor measures the pressure and stress of a situation (Yoels and Clair 1995:54). This is especially useful in contexts of marked status differences, where humor can be reflective of people's ease or unease with the situation. For people lower in the social hierarchy, laughter can form a conduit through which they can play with the social structure, turning it on its head. By making fun of Doctor Braulio's work ethic, Fabiola and the other women can redefine, albeit temporarily, their place within the social structure. He becomes the target of their criticism, and it is his behavior, rather than theirs, that is at fault. Through this type of humor, they have altered their status within the system: they are able to criticize those who ordinarily are in charge and who usually criticize them.

Humor is often one of the first victims of a difficult situation (Hart 2007): few revolutionaries can really be considered anything but humorless. Yet when one looks at how some of the least powerful members of society deal with the tremendous poverty, violence, or powerlessness in their lives, humor is frequently very present in their lives. For women suffering from breast cancer, humor plays the role of a coping mechanism, allowing them to find spirituality and hope in their lives (Johnson 2002). Among women living in a Brazilian *favela*, for instance, the humor is very dark, serving as a means to bring to light issues that would be considered impolite or shameful—such as the internalized racism coloring people's everyday lives (Goldstein 2003). Even refugees use jokes to poke fun at the direness of their situation as they list the many things that they lack in their lives (Rahul Oka, personal communication, March 25, 2011). Downe (1999) has shown in her work among sex workers in Costa Rica that the use of mocking and biting humor is a very effective weapon against the violence, discrimination, and inequities that the women face. The women's comfort with sexuality makes it possible for them to use sexual imagery to verbally attack the men (clients, politicians, and lawmakers) who oppress them.

Portraits of "The Mestizo"

Mexicans are humorous people—they tell jokes about all aspects of life. Jokes are commonplace and include everything from cutting political humor and jokes about political candidates, to gallows humor at the ravages of natural disasters such as earthquakes and hurricanes, to smart puns and witty language about swine flu, to ethnic jokes about rural or indigenous populations. Cantinflas is one of the most well-known comic creations: a beloved Chaplinesque movie character created in the 1930s representing Mexico's everyman. His "nonsensical [and] pun-riddled" discourses (Pilcher 2000:333) have given birth to the verb "*cantinflear*," to speak a lot but say little. La India Maria—the Indian Mary—another movie character with early beginnings in the 1970s, is a shambling and buffoonish caricature of the indigenous woman—ignorant, with an accent and hair in long plaits, and dressed in a mockery of indigenous clothes. Although she is the protagonist, she achieves success not by intelligence or even wiles, but through serendipity (De la Peña 1995)—and trouncing the city folk who stand in polar opposition to her rural, backwater roots. Her movies are marketed to the country's working class and provide an outlet for people to laugh at those even lower on the social ladder.

Storytelling among the Nahua is an art and a profession and is not something that just anyone can do. Humor was recurrently intertwined with the morals and life lessons embedded in the Nahua stories. Modesto, an elderly man with salt-and-pepper hair whose childlike joy of life was evident in his twinkling eyes, was a very adept and engrossing storyteller. He enjoyed regaling his listeners with funny tales, which he would relate with mischievous glee and laughter in his crinkly eyes. Sotero, from the neighboring village of Coatepec, was a professional storyteller who came over to Amatlán to visit relatives and would spend time recounting many stories with great good humor. I recorded several of Modesto's and Sotero's stories and realized that most of the underlying themes of the stories were about the underdog besting the oppressors and giving them their comeuppance.

While there are several recurring characters in many of the Nahua stories, there is a duo that appears more frequently and is an important depiction of the social structure of the region. This is the rabbit and coyote duo—a duo familiar to many in the global North as Uncle Remus's Brer Rabbit and Brer Fox. Coyote—or *coyotl* in Nahuatl—not only describes the predator but is also a term used pejoratively for the white man (see Sandstrom 1991), who is considered equally predatory. In these humorous stories, it is Conejo (Rabbit) who is the clever foil to Coyote's nefarious plans. The character of Coyote falls somewhere between stupid and canny—considered primarily a mischief maker (see Sandstrom 1991:69). As a representation of an outsider, especially a powerful outsider, he is always the butt of the jokes.[3]

Christie Davies (1990:315), in her analysis of ethnic humor around the world, demonstrates how such jokes "reflect the differential placing of ethnic groups within modern industrial societies." She argues that those represented as "stupid" are usually peasants or economically marginalized in some way, while those perceived as "canny" are not necessarily the most powerful but instead are those who have gained access to business or management through enterprise and calculation—such as trading groups (see also Oka 2008). I would counter that, at least in the case of the Coyote-Conejo stories, the coyote is not just a calculating outsider but is indeed a representation of the most powerful members of Mexican society who "exploit others when allowed" (Sandstrom 1991:69).

As do Keith Basso's portraits of "the Whiteman," the characterizations of the *mestizo* serve as a "conspicuous vehicle for conceptions that define and characterize what 'the Indian' is not" (Basso 1979:5). During Carnival in the Huasteca, men dress up as *mecos*, which are simultaneously representations of the underworld and satirized and mocked versions of the local *mestizos* (Sandstrom 1991:251; Provost 2004). The *mecos* at the Carnival celebrations I attended were primarily young men dressed up as women—some wearing miniscule miniskirts and diminutive tops likely borrowed from their sisters—with a bandana or a pink-faced mask covering their face. *Mecos* would dance and cavort (often lewdly) to very loud brass-band music in front of people's homes, refusing to leave until bribed by the householder to move on to the next victim. The humorous situations and characters that emerge in these encounters thus become vehicles for people to poke fun, in a hidden manner, at those who have historically oppressed them.

Haircuts for Chickens: Nahua Humor

The people in Amatlán laugh a lot. Their humor takes many forms: laughter at physical comedy—such as Esperanza giving one of her chickens a "haircut" to remove the many feathers that fell across its eyes; commiserative or understanding laughter at difficulties of life—the women merrily laughing about how every few years their chickens and turkeys die off in a bout of disease; and gentle double entendres about people's marital

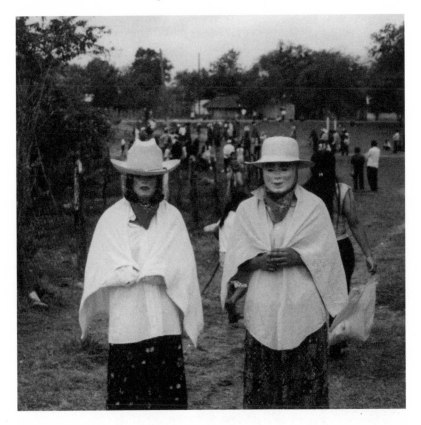

Figure 5.1. Mecos at Carnival

relationships and a lonely wife becoming *"fastidiada"* or bored when her husband is away.

For the women at the bakery co-operative, humor was a means to while away the time. One day, Lourdes joked that she planned to wear trousers, put on makeup, and wear a skimpy blouse and go dancing that night to the high school dance. Exuberantly miming the actions of dressing in teenage clothes and putting on makeup, Lourdes winked mischievously at her listeners. The women, for whom wearing trousers was unheard of, burst into fits of laughter, especially when she added, "Because I have no breasts I'm going to [stuff] in some balloons." The women retorted with several ribald comments about breast size, especially how hers would burst if someone squeezed them.

Much of the people's laughter revolved around ordinary life events. Any funny event that happened would soon be told to everyone in the village.

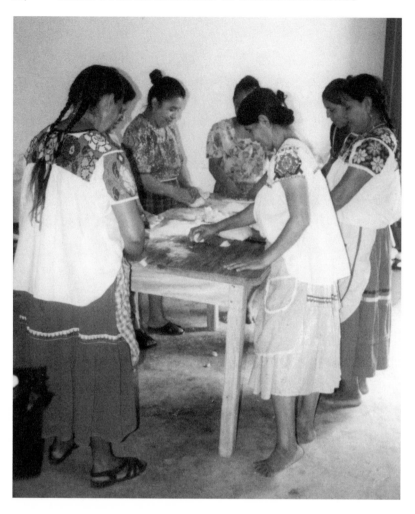

Figure 5.2. Making bread

When Teodora, an elderly woman, fell off her chair one evening, the story made the rounds across the village for many days. People would recount to each other with great glee how she had put her chair too close to the edge of the step and had fallen backward, and there she lay, with her legs up in the air. The usual greeting of "How is so and so at home?" was replaced with "Did you hear about how Teodora fell over and her legs stuck up in the air?" The fact that she was not well liked in the village certainly helped to fuel the laughter at her expense.

Laughter can also be a response to the strange. When Pentecostalism entered the area in the mid-1980s, many of the most disenfranchised of

Amatlán were the first to convert (Sandstrom 1991). Such conversion is a very common occurrence across the world, whereby people rework and reform their selves (Kray 2002). The beliefs and accompanying rituals that came alongside the conversion seemed bizarre to the rest of the villagers. Esperanza laughingly told me the following anecdote:

> Before, when they would carry out the *culto* they would go to the Temple and that man they call Cosme would stay outside.[4] And with a big club he would beat the ground. [He said] that he was frightening [away] the devil. And he would beat and beat [the ground] with that club, and he would go "fshshsh" "fshshsh," and he looked as though he was blind. We would laugh at him.

Esperanza paused a moment and then said, with a smile, "So he stopped doing that." The people's ridicule was a response to the seemingly bizarre behavior. It also drew a line between the Catholics and the Pentecostals and created a community and "collective consciousness" among the Catholics who shared in this laughter. Laughter in this case served a social function by "inviting those present to become close" (Coser 1959:172). Because of the laughter at their expense, which undermined the seriousness of their religious beliefs, the Pentecostals soon moved the public exorcising of the devil into the (laughter-proof) privacy of their homes.

The women do use humor to talk about things that would ordinarily be taboo (as Freud 2003 describes)—such as breast size in Fabiola's or Lourdes's jokes. They can use humor to defuse any social discomfort. When I was asked where my husband was and how he allowed me to come to the field alone, most people would laugh and then tease, "*Pero, te vas a fastidiar*" (But, you will get bored!). They would then follow up with a comment about how he would likely find someone else in my absence. Constanza asked me once if I was planning on having children. When I answered that I was finding it difficult to conceive, she retorted, "But how would you be able to [conceive] if you are here and [your husband] is there!" The humorous delivery of these statements makes the sexual subject matter palatable to all involved.

The women of Amatlán are full of laughter. Many of them are very adroit at recounting difficulties and making others laugh. Humor can be very effective at shifting the mood in a group. One morning a group of women spoke quietly about family planning, their somber faces showing some of the bewildering experiences many of them had gone through. Rosario piped up with her own concerns about family planning. She said,

"No I don't want to use the [IUD]; it scares me. They say it can get lost. And the men fear that it will get stuck [on their penis]. One of my sisters-in-law [said] that the [IUD] went all the way inside her, because she couldn't find it anymore." Smiling suddenly, she then said with a twinkle in her eye, "It did fall out of another sister-in-law. Her husband beat her and then he embraced her very hard [around the middle] and she said the IUD fell out. Yes, he embraced her and held her tightly and it fell out." As Rosario told this story, she mimed the man's violent embrace by holding her arms across her middle. Contorting her face she pushed out her hands to show how the IUD was squeezed out. Her use of facial expressions and mimicry, and the imagery she conjured up, made her listeners laugh out loud.

Altagracia, who lived across from Esperanza and Ildefonso, shared some of the heartbreaking events that had happened in her life. As she told these stories, she smiled often, to show that, though tragic, these events were not insurmountable. She said, "When we were young the men were just drunks. And they would fight like dogs, rolling around and beating each other. My father was like that." Standing up from her small chair and pacing around her small home, she began to mimic the actions of her father, pretending to slam doors and to throw things. Deepening her voice for effect, she said, "He would come in and roll up his sleeves and push open the door and he would shout at my mother that he was hungry. And when she would serve him he would take the plate [mimed holding plate up high and threateningly] and would want to beat my mother. I would take [the plate] away and he would just stare at me and he would pick up the cup and would also want to throw it at my mother." Smiling ruefully, she then said, "That's why I say that I grew up as a *borracha* [a drunk]. I didn't go to school and I don't know how to read or write. And I was still just a kid when the [missionaries] arrived." After recounting how her religious conversion was a turning point in her life, she continued:

> I got pregnant and could not give birth. I spent two nights [in labor] and the boy came out with a really long head. He didn't want to nurse or anything. He didn't cry. And we took him to a healer who said he would heal him, but as soon as he started [the healing ritual] the boy died. Then I had another one, but that one didn't want to nurse either. The *hermanos* [members of the Pentecostal faith] said that if I had faith in God, the [boy] would be saved. So they came and they prayed and read the Bible and they said I had to have faith in God. And soon the boy began to nurse. He had been healed.

As with Goldstein's *favela* inhabitants, many of these stories are ways for the listeners to make structural sense of these problems. Women also use humor to make visible the ways—often ignored—by which their lives are constrained. When recounting "jocular gripes" (Coser 1959:173) of their interactions with life, the laughter and giggles that ensue ease the women's frustration and ask the listeners to sympathize and "look what my life is like" or "look what I had to put up with today." Commiseration and comradeship are natural effects of this laughter. The humor is "an expression of the collective experience of the participants, and receives response only from those who share common concerns" (Coser 1959:173). In turn, such laughter embodies undercurrents of disobedience to the larger system; it is a way for the women to thumb their noses at those in power—clinicians, politicians, or men—from the safety of their home.

"You all know it harms you, yet you keep on doing it": *Jokes in the Medical Setting*

Some of the medical personnel—particularly the physicians—have established a joking relationship with their patients. In such relationships between two people, one is expected to tease or poke fun at the other, who, in turn, is not meant to take offense. In the case of the physicians and patients, it is an asymmetrical relationship wherein it is the former who tease the latter (Radcliffe-Browne 1940). (Only in private do the patients joke about the physician.) While on most occasions the physicians' interactions with the patients were professional and formal, there were instances where the physicians would relax and tease and joke with their patients. These jokes were a variant on the insistence present in all the medical interactions with patients. I observed several occasions where the physicians would tease the patients about a variety of things, including their weight, dietary habits, or following *autocuidado*—all aimed at obtaining patient compliance. "You are just lazy, nothing is actually hurting you" was a common, albeit unkind, joke.

Most jokes aimed at the women revolved around aspects of the women's lifestyle that were perceived to be problematic in some way. In a sense, culturally taboo topics do not generally exist in medicine, as the discipline is considered to be apart from culture. Hence physicians do not usually feel much discomfort talking about topics that would be culturally taboo among Mexicans or among women—such as sexuality. Yet there is a cultural divide between the groups, and so physicians likely use the jokes as a means to mediate between their and the women's cultures in a less direct way (Freud 2003).

Research into the use of humor in clinical settings shows that humor and jokes can integrate or differentiate the participants in the joke (Yoels and Clair 1995). Under certain circumstances, jokes can bring about a sense of collectivity, a unity. The laughter and humor of the women listening to Fabiola's story can act as a means of integrating and differentiating (Yoels and Clair 1995:49) and may have served to blur the status lines between them and the physician. (As I showed above, humor can serve to strengthen the women collectively and invert the social structure.) But under other circumstances, particularly when the joke travels down the social structure and where there is already a tension in the social structure because of inequalities of status, the joke simply broadens the fissures existent between the participants. As an example of this expansion of social differences, one finds that it is jokes that mock the people's customs that cut the most deeply, separating the joker from the object of the joke. For instance, rather than a strong, Western-style handshake, where the whole hand is gripped, people in this region typically greet each other by touching only the fingertips of the other person's hand. It is a very soft and gentle greeting. Yet in a biomedical setting, it looks out of place, and when Doctora Felipa was greeted in this manner by a patient, she snickered and said, "These people's [funny] customs."

Yoels and Clair (1995) demonstrate how the historical contexts of status and power profoundly shape the way that the joking interactions take place. The history of indigenous and *mestizo* relations of this region has created a definite distance between these groups, which is mirrored by the presence of humor in the people's encounters. Thus "these people's [funny] customs" not only becomes a scornful comment in response to an encounter between physician and patient but also reflects the almost insurmountable social divide between the parties. Through this mocking phrase, the division between physician and patient, powerful and powerless, us and them, becomes all the more emphasized. One may imagine that any patient hearing such a comment from his or her physician would be unable to retort in any effective, public way. This inability to counter would feed back into the disempowerment felt by patients in these contexts.

In the clinical settings in the region, the physicians were usually the ones to instigate a humorous situation or make a joke about a patient or the situation. Physicians are much more likely to be at ease in these circumstances, and so humor can simply flow within their conversations with patients. Fabiola probably felt much more comfortable poking fun at the physician's work habits because the conversation took place in Amatlán, as opposed to at the clinic, which often has a silencing effect on the women. The targets of humor are very rarely socially higher than the person who utters the joke but rather are of lower status (Yoels and Clair 1995), and though perhaps the physicians are not aware of it, the targets are unlikely to be able to publicly rebuff the humor in any satisfactory way.

Most of the jokes flow from the physicians to the patients. The nurses' role is often as gatekeeper to the physician and the medical center, and as such, they are much more serious about health care and rarely joke with their patients. Their role in monitoring all aspects of each patient's health and filling out paperwork left less room to joke with the people in the clinic or hospital. They had to manage a large number of patients and obtain health care for them.

Nurse Juliana at Tepatepec worked on a daily basis and often seemed harassed. Her primary role of manager of people's health means that she uses any method possible to obtain people's compliance—from teasing to outright criticism. She was particularly critical of women's family planning and related health. When Matilde, a mother of four in her mid-thirties, went in for her annual check-up, Juliana immediately brought out Matilde's *cartilla de planificación familiar*—her family-planning card. After weighing and measuring her, Juliana asked her what her diet consisted of. She then told Matilde to "stop eating salt, because that swells up your legs. The veins become inflamed with the [contraceptive] pill. If you want we can look into the injection. You should not eat *chile*, fats, soft drinks." Turning to the rest of the women gathered at the clinic, she said loudly, "And [all of] you know that they are bad for you yet you keep on doing it!" While Juliana's intention was to rebuke, Matilde simply laughed quietly. She was joined by other women, who tittered at the nurse's castigation. Most of them had been the butt of such comments in past interactions, and in many ways, their laughter was commiserative.

These interactions do not mean that the nurses are cold; indeed, they are often much more nurturing and warm to the people than the physicians are. It is evident that the nurses at these medical centers tend to be better liked than the physicians, as shown by the fact that at the end of the school year, they frequently receive a stream of requests to be *madrinas*—godmothers—to graduating students. Nurses only infrequently joked with their patients. On those rare occasions that they did use humor, the jokes took the form of teasing, such as when Juliana joked with a young girl whose birthday it was to ask her parents for a cake as a present. One of the women listening to this responded by loudly saying that there was no money for such frivolities. Such a blunt statement about their poverty caused the rest of the women to burst into laughter.

Vera Robinson (1970), in a short article on humor in medical situations, argues that humor used by nurses serves to promote harmony in social relations and to diminish discomfort and awkwardness. She points out that humor can be also useful to facilitate learning—by developing warmth between people, relieving stress, releasing anger, and avoiding people's pain and discomfort. It is mostly in this context—as a learning tool—that the Ixhuatlán nurses used humor, especially as they managed the *pláticas* of Oportunidades to encourage the women to develop better *autocuidado* and mothering techniques.

Juliana was one of the few nurses I saw tease her patients on one or two occasions. One day she was manning her desk and attending to various patients one after the other. One of the first sets of patients that day was a man and a woman, both of whom looked as though they were in their fifties. The man came up to Juliana's desk and told her, "My wife will be the patient [today]." Juliana brought the file out and gave it a quick glance to check the woman's and her family's general health and information. She turned to the woman and asked her for her age, holding her pen expectantly over her paperwork. The woman replied quietly that she did not know. Juliana looked up at her quickly with a disbelieving face and then just as quickly looked down at the chart. She said, "It is 52." To the world at large she then said, "She does not know." Turning back to the woman, she said slowly, as though speaking to a child, "Remember that each year you add *one* more year [to your age]." Hunching her shoulders, the woman cast down her eyes in embarrassment. While Juliana's aim was to tease the woman and help her to remember her age, her tone of voice—and her informing the other patient about the woman's ignorance—might also have been designed to embarrass her and show the differences in status between them. This, however, might not necessarily have been the nurse's intention but was rather simply the emerging situation.

Humor fills the spaces between the body and the self (Yoels and Clair 1995). It can create a more tangible connection between them. This is especially the case for clinicians, as they are primarily concerned with the body, while the patients are usually concerned with both their body (what they are feeling regarding their ailment) and their self (how they are feeling about it). Humor can therefore create a social bond between the participants in that interaction, as it brings the participants together. A joke about a patient's individual body and what that person is going through can become a reflection of society at large (Lock and Scheper-Hughes 1987). The humor embedded in the interactions between physician and patient not only reflect certain ills of society, but they might also serve to break down some of the divisions between the participants—albeit temporarily—and connect the person's self to the person making the humorous comment (see Yoels and Clair 1995).

Laughing While It Hurts: Gallows Humor

While most of the jokes emanating from the clinicians seem to be primarily inoffensive—though always containing the core of correction and development of the women's lives—there are some that extend into gallows humor. In gallows humor, the jokes revolve around life-threatening or painful situations in an effort to alleviate tension. Yoels and Clair (1995) show that humor can also be used to create separation between people in an interaction. Patients can distance themselves from the encounter by using humor to protect their selves—their individual bodies.

One evening in early 2004, Esperanza and I were sitting on the front veranda of her house. Her veranda is a lovely place to sit in the cool evenings, as one can see the world pass by while sitting in a lightly breezy area. As we sat, several people passed by and greeted us with "We are going [home]," "We are going that way," and "We are going to the chapel." While we sat enjoying the gentle breeze, a shiny, black, four-wheel-drive pickup truck drove up and parked in front of the house. Though several families in the village have pickups, most are old, second-hand rejects from the United States that are brought down to Mexico to be sold at excessively high prices to rural Mexicans. This was not one of those cars. Though I did not recognize the man who emerged, one could tell from the car and his appearance that he was not an indigenous farmer. He was Doctor Fermín, a well-established *mestizo* physician from Ixhuatlán who was seeking endorsements and votes for his campaign for municipal president. He had come to talk with Ildefonso, who at that time happened to be the village *agente*, to try to convince him not only to vote for him but also to get him to encourage the other villagers to do likewise. Ildefonso, who embodies Plato's ideal of a reluctant ruler, dislikes politics of any sort and thus simply was politely noncommittal to the man's entreaties.

As politics of this sort are a man's domain, the men sat on one end of the veranda while Esperanza, Tito, and I moved our chairs to the other end. We were not invited to be part of any of the conversation. Nonetheless, Esperanza provided a glimpse into the social interactions of Doctor Fermín when she turned to me and began to recount, slightly conspiratorially, an experience she went through over twenty years ago. This experience perfectly illustrates gallows humor—and how humor often breaks down if not all parties share the joke. As she told the story, she spoke quietly, clasped her hands in her lap, and cast her eyes downward. She often held this pose while recounting difficult memories.

Esperanza said that she had been suffering from horrible headaches and went to Ixhuatlán to see Doctor Fermín. He plied her with medicines and told her she had to go back to him over and over again. But nothing helped. She said that the last time she was there,

> I was lying inside [his office] and he told me I was going to die and he wanted me to get out. He forced me to get out. I wanted to rest my head and then leave, but he pushed me out. [He said] that he did not want me to die there. He did not attend to me anymore. That is why I have told my husband not to support him.

At those words, she looked up and laughed. Her change in tone was surprising, especially after delivering the story so somberly. She exclaimed, "That is why I don't believe in doctors. They know nothing!" She then compared this physician to El Doctor Gastón—a practically herculean physician who has a private practice in Ixhuatlán and who everyone holds up as the paragon of goodness—and said that he was integral in improving the health of one of her sons, even going so far as to give him the medicine for free. The image of the good physician was promptly broken, however, when she added, "He also wanted to be [municipal] president [a few years ago]. I fed him when he came [to campaign]. Many supported him. But he found out who had not supported him and now he charges them a lot [more] when they go to his clinic."

Doctor Fermín's words to Esperanza on that night open up an interesting array of possibilities. On the one hand, he might have been deadly serious, tossing Esperanza out of his office because he did not want to deal with her. On the other, he might have simply been using gallows humor to lighten a woebegone situation: he was not making any headway in curing her headaches and chose to poke fun at the situation by making a joke about its direness, accompanying Esperanza out of his office, telling her not to die on him.

Gallows humor is likely to work best when all parties involved actually understand the reason for the joke and are also of similar status, not where one party is dependent on the other for something—in this case good health. Gallows humor can, thus, be dangerous for physicians to use as it serves to distance themselves from the patient. Such humor is exclusionary—someone is the insider telling the joke, possessing more information about the situation than the outsider, who is often the butt of the joke (and is thus unlikely to appreciate the humor at their expense) (Berger et al. 2004). This form of humor is morbid and meant to terrify. To a gravely ill patient, such as Esperanza, who had struggled to make her way to Ixhuatlán (which at that time was about a four-hour walk across the countryside, and required crossing several streams and a large river), and who had suffered debilitating headaches, such words—even if meant in jest—were not a laughing manner. Under the circumstances, she took those words as harsh reality, where the physician cared nothing for her needs and simply tossed her out when he could not deal with her anymore.

Medical examinations (even routine ones) are usually moments of anxiety for patients. While for physicians these encounters are routine and part and parcel of their daily lives, such is not the case for patients. Thus patients might be more prone to misinterpreting the interaction between themselves and their physician and be perhaps not very likely to find humor in the situation—especially if they are the object of the joke (Yoels and Clair 1995). This is especially the case for the indigenous populations served at the clinics in the area of Amatlán, as going to the physician is rarely routine. People either go to the clinic for their once-a-year requirement through Oportunidades or because they have an illness or medical emergency. Hence "routine" is far from their minds. Humor can thus be perceived to be more "aggressive" in their eyes than in those of the physician.

In Esperanza's story can be found a variety of features typical of the relationship between women and the physicians—as well as the construction of subjects through the use of humor. Esperanza felt wronged by Doctor Fermín by not being treated as she deserved—neither for the headaches nor as a woman. While she still did not find humor in the situation years later, she was able to laugh at her opposition to his political aspirations. The fact that Esperanza did not die meant that her dislike for this particular physician simply increased. Her vehement statement about physicians knowing nothing shows the disdain she feels toward Doctor Fermín—and the medical profession in general. She now fights back through covert means, such as convincing Ildefonso not to vote for him.

Turning to Doctor Fermín's presence at Ildefonso and Esperanza's house on the evening in question, one can see that, at least in his case, he did not remember (or place much importance on) the past interaction between him and Esperanza. Perhaps this is an indication of the fact that he was making a joke on that day long ago and did not notice the effect it had on his patient. In a darker—and perhaps truer—interpretation of the interactions between the elite classes and the indigenous people of the region, he probably neither remembered that particular interaction nor connect a lone indigenous woman from twenty years ago to the present-day wife of a man whose vote he now sought.[5]

Cutting the Flesh: Grim Gallows Humor

In the medical setting, the women rarely relaxed; instead they would often be very stiff, barely speaking, and very compliant. They took the word of the medical staff to be the truth, and thus when the physicians told them that they would carry out certain procedures, it was not received as idle joking but as grim reality.

Dulce's case is probably the most poignant example of this grimness. She is in her late twenties and has five children. Her seeming stubbornness regarding contraception was frequently a source of annoyance to the staff at the clinic. During one visit, one of the male physicians jokingly scolded her for having too many children and "always being pregnant." He said to her in exasperation, "I will forcibly operate on you, even if it is right here and with a knife." Though his intention was to joke and tease her, it was a very chilling example of the power that rests in the physicians' hands.

What was interesting about this interaction was that while the women tittered politely at this joke when they were at the clinic, when they recounted it to each other later, once they were back in Amatlán, they did so with much laughter. All the women have been at the receiving end of frustrated comments of that sort at some point, and thus their laughter created a bond between them and was commiserative and showed that "we are all in this boat." The women engaged in gallows humor through laughing at this joke (which in itself was gallows humor). Hart (2007), in her analysis of humor and social movements, shows that gallows humor is used by many to psychologically escape from the unalterable. The self-deprecating nature of such jokes "serve[s] to bolster fellowship among oppressed or marginalized ethnic groupings" (6). And while Hart states that a joke that is funny in these contexts fails to be so when told by those in power, the physician's joke that he was going to cut into Dulce's flesh is an example of a comment that emerges from the powerful and then is reinterpreted and humorized by the marginalized.

What is often evident in the clinics and hospitals is the asymmetrical relationship between a *mestizo* physician and an indigenous woman. In most of these encounters, the women have no choice but to accept the comments leveled at them, which reflect and replicate the dominant structures present throughout Mexican society (Maternowska 2006:78; see also Nazar Beutel-spacher et al. 2003). These structures contrast a marginalized, uneducated, indigenous, rural woman on the one hand, and a dominant, educated, *mestizo*, urban person (male or female) on the other. As I have shown throughout this book, the dominant structures of Mexican society expect a certain type of behavior from its citizens. These expectations are particularly stringent for low-income, rural, or indigenous mothers, and even more so for someone who is all three.

"El Pinche Doctor": *The Many Roles of Humor*

Within the women's laughter exists an opposition to the difficulties they face in their life. Their good humor and ability to laugh at the lack of medical care, at poor treatment at medical centers, and at the (albeit infrequent) retorts some women make to the physicians' jokes at their expense demonstrate their ability to mock certain aspects of their lives. This sort of laughter is by no means overt resistance. They rarely called the physician's words into question but instead laughed politely at his jokes and then privately laughed about other entirely different matters—particularly by making fun of the clinic and its staff. Humor allows them to question the oppression of their lives and to bring to light the strong discrepancy between the imagery of the idealized behavior they are meant to follow and the gritty reality of their lives. Through their laughter they can also turn the tables on the clinic and point out its various inefficiencies.

Donna Goldstein (2003), in her work on women in a Brazilian *favela*, shows how humor is used by women to deal with the violence that they experience in their living and working conditions in a society where class distinctions and poverty are ever present. Humorous stories, jokes, and retellings of difficult situations, such as the rape of two young women, become ways for the women to cope with domestic violence and female victimization. Laughter was a particularly useful tool for the women to discuss the role of men in their lives and to "reveal a great deal of suffering that otherwise would have remained silent" (265). These acts of humor are the hidden transcripts (Scott 1990) of people's resistance. They are not public and thus can easily be dismissed, yet their covert nature is what makes them all the more effective as weapons of resistance for the least powerful members of a society.

Humor provides the context to understand the daily structuring of class, ethnicity, gender, and violence wherein these jokes are "embedded and entangled" (Goldstein 2003: 273). While understanding the context allows one to "get" the joke, the "humor both masks and reveals . . . the very structures and hierarchies on which the humor depends" (273). The women are not merely passive victims of the structures "of domination that construct their lives" (273). Seeing such hostile humor as cathartic, Freud (2003) states that it allows one "to turn to good account those ridiculous features in our enemy that the presence of opposing obstacles would not let us utter aloud or consciously" (98). It ultimately becomes a form of resistance to difficult situations. As do the sex workers in Downe's study (1999) and the *favela* women in Goldstein's, the women of Amatlán "enact and reproduce these structures" because they live them. They simultaneously "strenuously and creatively resist them" (Goldstein 2003:273). As Goldstein puts it, after having done all they can do, the only thing left for them is laughter; it becomes "laughter out of place" (272).

For most of people, politicians represented what was wrong with the state of affairs in Ixhuatlán. They knew that "these people just come with promises and then do nothing," as Alcides, an elderly man in Amatlán, said loudly as he heckled a campaigning politician, banging his walking stick angrily on the ground for effect. Despite this knowledge, people always hoped that they could reap as much as they could from campaigning politicians, knowing that once the politicians entered office they would receive nothing more.

Gloria took advantage of politicians' "largesse" during one campaign. She accepted a concrete oven solely because she was also promised construction gravel, which she sorely needed. Much to her consternation, she never received any gravel. Women were often enticed to go to political rallies with promises of *despensas*—food baskets—and other home products, such as buckets or plastic containers. Emma and her daughter Jacqueline went to one rally during an extremely hot day in May where women had been promised a sizeable *despensa*. On their return, they recounted that the extreme heat had caused a child to succumb to sunstroke and that a second one had been barely saved from a similar fate. Emma then added as an afterthought as she wiped perspiration from her face, "They promised us a *despensa*, but at the end [of the event] they only gave us a sandwich and a water!" Her face then broke into a large smile, and she and Jacqueline burst into laughter. For both of them, the horror of the child's death combined with the indignity of the political machinations left them with little else to do but laugh at the injustice of it all.

Esperanza recounted a similar story, saying, "[Politicians] only come and they tell us how they will help us and everything that they'll do but they don't even listen to us. . . . The current [municipal] president even came with his wife and promised us that he would help and so we all voted for him. His wife said she would come with *despensas*." She added, laughing scornfully, "But they never gave us anything!" Then she said, "Like when I had to buy medication for my son [Adrian] the medicine was 300 pesos for a week's worth. The teacher gave me a paper and told me to go to the [municipal presidency] to ask them for monetary support. [He said] that they do have money [and might give me] 'at least one thousand pesos.' But they didn't give me any and they even asked me why I didn't work to make that money." Laughing at the politician's stinging comments about her inability to make ends meet, she concluded bitterly, "So I didn't even give them the piece of paper and I didn't go back!"

Esperanza's and Emma's use of laughter was a means of making sense of the structural violence they experienced. While it is expected that politicians will lie, most people still retain the hope that the long Mexican tradition of political patronage and clientelism will be honored. When they are invariably disappointed, humor becomes a salve to comfort their frustration. As Hong (2010:31) writes in his analysis of humor in German-occupied Denmark, humor allows the tellers to navigate the difficulties that they face and to cope with "a world [they] cannot control or fully understand."

Humor also helps to reduce conflict (Berger et al. 2004; Hong 2010). Rather than the women becoming upset at the absence of medical personnel at the clinic or at the indignities they face at the hands of politicians, they laugh about the situation. Laughter becomes a way for them to defuse any anger or hostility they might feel. By sharing their laughter with other women in the village, the women create a sense of collectivity.

The physicians and nurses also use humor to deal with the frustrations they encounter as practitioners in marginalized areas. They are frustrated with many of the behaviors of their patients, as in the interaction between Matilde and Nurse Juliana I described earlier. They also are clearly bored by repeating the same instructions daily to populations that they see as willfully noncompliant (see Maternowska 2006). While the clinicians do count some changes in people's behaviors as small victories—as when Juliana proudly told me that in the time she has worked in Tepatepec, people have become more conscientious about bathing—their daily interactions with patients tend to highlight the uphill battle they face. Almost every time I was at the clinics and hospitals, the staff was scolding someone for not having a good diet or not using family planning. After a long day of seeing patient after patient, Doctora Felipa turned to me in frustration and said, "It is just that they do not want to develop. They are this way because they want to be." This comment illustrates the many frustrations felt by the staff, and by disclosing her thoughts to me, an obvious outsider, Doctora Felipa is able to share her annoyance while simultaneously defusing it.

Even support staff fall prey to the frustrations. Azalea, a *mestiza* woman in her early thirties, with big brown eyes and blue eye shadow, who was always meticulously dressed in skirts and blouses and beautiful stone jewelry to match, worked in human resources at the hospital in Llano. She told me about a frustrating interaction with a young patient she had just recently experienced:

> This girl came in who wanted a pregnancy test, but she already had a little tummy. . . . She insisted and insisted on the test so we did a blood test. Later on she asks me how it came out and I told her, "Look, child, well, you are pregnant." But we did not understand each other and she kept on saying she wanted to know. And she stubbornly wanted to know. Sometimes one cannot understand them. It turns out that what she wanted to know was who the father was. . . . But I told her, "Child, you cannot [know that] just with the blood [test]" as you need to know the father's blood type and all. But she was adamant that she wanted to know. She was already six months [pregnant] and only thirteen!

Though Azalea told the story with a serious face, showing her frustration, as she concluded, she sighed and laughed out loud. This laughter tempered her frustration. Her words show a clear divide between herself, as someone in possession of accurate knowledge, and "them"—who reproduce young, have too many children, and do not understand even seemingly straightforward concepts such as paternity testing. By laughing, she could defuse her frustration instead of allowing it to fester, thereby affect-ing her work and interaction with problematic patients.

The clinicians see these problematic behaviors as symptomatic of the intractable nature of the indigenous peasantry. Similar to the upper-middle-class Haitian doctors in Catherine Maternowska's (2006) research at a family-planning center in Port au Prince, this perception conforms to the dominant class's expectations about "appropriate behavior toward the poor" (78). The perceived disobedience of their patients only reinforces medical practitioners' frustration with them, and this frustration is con-verted into humor as a coping mechanism for themselves. They use hu-mor to make light of the matter. They poke fun at the women, joke about some of the medical procedures they will perform, and tease women about their removal from Oportunidades. While from the outside—and from the women's perspective—such jokes border on the cruel, for the physicians they are a means to reduce their frustration as well as to pos-sibly chivy their patients into obedience and compliance.

It is the asymmetrical relationship between the participants that makes humor in the clinical context troublesome. Many of the women will laugh in response to difficulties encountered at the clinic and, in doing so, are op-posing the clinical setting and its precepts. They laugh at the physicians and nurses, but only in private and in the company of other women from their community. The laughter is rarely open in the presence of the authorities—the open laughter at the physician in Fabiola's story is unusual and was likely because the physician was in *their* territory rather than them being in his. But because the women do not laugh openly at the medical orders and practices in the clinical setting, they are not truly resisting or disobeying the system. Their private laughs are outlets for their frustrations and anger. By laughing, they defuse these feelings. Their laughter simply serves as a means for them to feel better, as nothing actually changes when they laugh.

Laughter has been analyzed as a weapon of the weak for resistance (Scott 1985). Scott sees disenfranchised people using covert and hidden forms of resistance in their daily lives to counter some of the indignities they suffer at the hands of those in power. In his view, peasants continually resist the domination of the elite classes by small acts of opportunistic opposition. Abu-Lughod (1990) warns against romanticizing resistance and instead advocates for its use as a diagnostic of power. Narrating the lives of Bedouin women, she describes four types of resistance—women sharing secrets and covering for each other against the world of men; women resisting an unwanted marriage; women using lyric poetry to subvert moral codes that perpetuate unequal power systems; and women using jokes and sexually irreverent discourse to ridicule the men's moral codes that oppress them. Yet as Abu-Lughod states, even these forms of resistance are disappearing as the Bedouin become increasingly connected to broader forces of modernization and enmeshed "in new sets of power relations of which they are scarcely aware" (50). She adds that resistance reveals much about the "historically changing relations of power" in which populations are enmeshed as they become increasingly incorporated into the mainstream (Abu-Lughod 1990:41).

Ahearn (2001:115) cautions that conflation of agency with resistance is problematic, as "oppositional agency is only one of many forms of agency." She adds, quoting Arlene MacLeod, that women, though often subordinate, "always play an active part that goes beyond the dichotomy of victimization/acceptance, a dichotomy that flattens out a complex and ambiguous agency in which women accept, accommodate, ignore, resist, or protest—sometimes all at the same time" (Ahearn 2001:116). Despite the many considerations of agency, power, and resistance that have shown humor as an act of resistance, I am not convinced that what is occurring when the Amatlán women's laugh is actually resistance. I see their laughter more as part of their larger habitus, reproductive or otherwise, where they are predisposed to behave in ways that reproduce the system of inequalities they live in.

Humor in itself never actually changes people's circumstances. The women's laughter rarely helped the women to solve their lack of agency. Instead, it functioned as a means to defuse their irritation or anger, which would consequently reduce their opposition to their treatment and any conflict they might engage in. As Hart (2007:7) shows, "humor may even lessen discontent among the oppressed, which might inhibit the mobilization into action." In this regard, jokes are often viewed as safety valves that remove people's outright anger and channel it into a more benign outlet—in the same way that Carnival functions. Hong (2010) points out that laughing or jeering at something or someone that causes one trouble might provide emotional satisfaction; and doing so in private means that there are no actual consequences—positive or negative—of outright confrontation. The people's imaginary power remains imaginary, and even if they feel good while laughing, the laughter has no real social or political effect. Paradoxically, rather than being a means to resist, laughter results in making the women even more compliant and obedient.

If the women are obedient, they will not have any agency and thus will have no way of actually effecting change in the policies that circumscribe them. Aurora, one of the kindergarten teachers in Amatlán, was quite critical of the way that the women are expected to attend to the rules and how they are affected by the consequences if they do not. She often told the women not to be so docile and to fight for what they want and need. While much of the women's docility comes from their discomfort with upsetting the status quo—the people from this area are particularly polite and courteous—much of it probably originates from their laughter.

I witnessed only a few women openly contradict or even defy the physicians. Most women would listen quietly to the instructions, and even if they eventually did what they pleased, they rarely questioned the information or the tone in which it was imparted. Lourdes was one of the few women who did speak her mind. She did so both in the clinical setting and in the privacy of her home. Her assertiveness likely originated from her belief that she was "like a doctor" and knew just as much as physicians and other clinicians. Indeed, she felt she was better than any physician as she had received the gift of healing from God, a claim none of the physicians could make. Because of her training and confidence, she never held back on her opinions of the physicians. She was one of the few women who used profanities, referring to the physician in Tepatepec as "*el pinche doctor,*" the damn doctor, on several occasions. To echo MacLeod, in this statement Lourdes is simultaneously opposing, resisting, and bowing down to the realities she faces—while she can rail at the physician, she knows that she is dependent on his good graces to remain a part of Oportunidades.

The mocking, sarcastic attitude of the clinicians is not unique to Amatlán or to any of the hospitals or clinics of the area. It is instead a manifestation of the medical authority that has been recognized by various authors and researchers across the world. Maternowska (2006) describes the many nasty jibes that poor Haitian women face at the hands of clinicians at a family-planning clinic. Castro (2004) shows the ways that Mexican physicians strenuously advocate for low-income women's sterilization and how they express dismay when women refuse. Lazarus (1997) describes how women's knowledge about their own bodies is subsumed under the physician's authoritative knowledge emerging from the information garnered from the fetal monitor. Scheper-Hughes (2002) recognizes the "bad faith" of physicians in Brazil who substitute medicines for food for their extremely malnourished patients. While a reliance on medical and technical solutions to the women's poverty and high number of children exists throughout Mexico, such reliance among clinicians in Ixhuatlán does include at least some acknowledgment of the larger structures that create these situations.

The effect of the stern joking persona that the clinicians establish to deal with their patients—by obliging the "respect that they deserve" in Nurse Juliana's words—provokes a response in the women. The women see the interactions and jokes as inappropriate; they see them as stern finger wagging and as an indictment of their mothering and of their reproductive habitus. The women react to accusations by accessing their own humor and by laughing at their marginality. The alternating structure of humor displayed by many of the women's stories—the recounting difficult memories (loss of a child, mistreatment by physicians or politicians, domestic violence, and so on) followed by quick, pithy comments and laughter—was a very normal pattern for the women and men of the region.

While the purpose of humor can be to strengthen bonds and play with social interactions, in its secondary purpose of defusing anger, it reduces people's impetus to revolt. As Hong (2010) discusses, laughter creates acquiescence. So while women laugh in response to problems, they become less upset. This, in turn, allows them to continue their lives—as they can acknowledge that things will rarely change. This acknowledgment makes them calm, and their calmness decreases their need to complain. By refraining from complaining, they continue to be compliant. This becomes the greatest irony of their laughter. They laugh at the constraints of the modern world, and through their ensuing obedience, they become increasingly moldable by the state into ideal modern mothers and citizens.

Conclusion

"I nurture them because I love them"

A FEW YEARS AFTER RETURNING FROM AMATLÁN, WHILE I WAS GOING through my field notes in preparing my book manuscript, I came across these words from Cristina. We had spent much of that day talking about her motherhood, her children, and Oportunidades. One of the questions I asked her was, "What happens if you do not follow the rules?" Cristina earnestly replied, "They take away your Oportunidades. As a responsible mother one has to take one's child to the clinic. They would take [the money] away if we were irresponsible. We take [the money] away from ourselves." She sat back in her chair with a self-satisfied smile playing on her face; Cristina knew that she was not one of the irresponsible mothers she was describing. I probed with another question, "What do they say at the clinic if you do not go regularly?" Her answer once again showed the internalization of compliance and responsibility. She said, "They report you. . . . There is someone there to supervise and check. The doctor and nurse are not to blame [for the money being taken away] but rather the patient herself." Cristina's notions of responsibility and irresponsibility regarding motherhood align with those of the state, and she has internalized the expectations of obedience.

The women I met are good mothers; their actions speak to the love they have for their children. They invest emotionally in their children from the moment they are pregnant—and afterward they express their love through a physical nurturance of extended breastfeeding, bed sharing, and lengthy carrying and hugging. "I nurture them because I love them" was a common refrain for the women. All these actions (conscious and unconscious) form part of their reproductive and mothering habitus. These women have certain mothering dispositions that they have been inculcated in from previous generations—and in turn they inculcate their own (female) children into these dispositions. In their interaction with a rapidly changing world, these dispositions change: some remain, while others "engender both aspirations and practice" (Bourdieu 1977:77). As Sulkunin would put it, the women's habitus is constantly being formed in their daily practices, by their producing and using their systems of meaning (Harker 1984:120).

But these mothers are repeatedly told that they are not, in fact, good mothers. They are told by Oportunidades that they will be good mothers only if they follow the conditions; they are informed that the only good mothering is the mainstream, modern, and nonindigenous form; and they are reminded that if their children are not perfect future citizens, the fault lies with their own poor mothering. During Mexico's dance with eugenics and nationalism, mothers have been historically identified simultaneously as shapers and destroyers of the nation. Efforts—through health campaigns, media ads, soap opera spots, and puericulture—have been designed to curb any problems and indoctrinate good behavior.

Humor becomes a tool for the women to manage their overly monitored lives. Esperanza, Cristina, Lourdes, Frida, and Alicia used good humor and many laughs to figure out their powerlessness. Humor also allowed them to regain some semblance of control and laugh at life as women and mothers, though most times, humor was just that—laughter at the funny things in life. These women are simply living their lives—at times they are agents, while at others they are not. The absurdity present in many of their interactions with the state apparatus became visible through their laughter. Their mirth defused any wrath, yet in practicing mirth, their compliance was assured. No righteous outrage emerged from these women; instead their laughs calcified their position within the domestic, unnoticed domain.

As I wrote this book, I frequently despaired at the gloomy picture I was drawing—of a hopeless situation where indigenous mothers are oppressed by the very system intent on their empowerment. I was told by family members and friends how negative this view was, as they questioned whether a program aimed at developing the welfare of women and children could possibly be that bad.

I found myself bending over backward in my effort to find positive attributes of the program. There is no denying that there are many good things that Oportunidades has brought to the community—an increase in cash flow, a rise in high school graduation, an improvement in children's and women's health, and an increase in women's knowledge of contraceptive methods. An associated benefit is the establishment of the Universidad Veracruzana Intercultural in Ixhuatlán (the UVI), which has allowed these high school graduates to pursue a locally relevant (and, it is hoped, also nationally relevant) university education.[1] Mothers are trusted with large amounts of cash, potentially leading to their domestic empowerment.

But time and again, I would come back to the women's concerns. "Your body is no longer the same," said Juana, referring to the effects of the medical treatment of their wombs and reproductive bodies. The women's bewilderment at the way the clinicians treated them could not be dismissed lightly. The women wistfully spoke about how "there used to be more children," perceiving an emptiness in the village. They expressed a bittersweet sense of loss through their participation in modernizing their motherhood.

The enrolled mothers have to constantly renegotiate their knowledge and agency, a process that erodes not only their former knowledge and power system but also the measure of their worth. In the village, they are strong, independent, autonomous women who know who they are. Even though they have problems in their own lives, they have the knowledge and often the means to solve them. They do this by accessing their networks and arranging the solution to their problems. This perception of themselves, however, changes at the intersection with development, where they see themselves as the development and biomedical forces see them: as a priori failures and as poor, ignorant, indigenous women with no hope unless they comply with the conditions of the Oportunidades program. One of the physician's words illustrates this situation well:

> People are lazy. They don't bother to use the resources they have available. It is easier to ask for beans, fry them up, and [eat] *chile* and *tortilla* and such. Lately I insist a lot, [telling them], "Hey, look, you have *nopales* there.[2] Wash them, boil them, throw in some egg. There is rice, cut up some corn. And in your own *milpa* there are squashes [and] *chayotes*.[3] Dice them and toss them into the rice [and eat them with] the beans and *tortillas*." Things change that way. People are just not used to using their resources; it's terrible. For instance, I tell them "look, instead of buying some *tostes* and some Sabritas [a potato chip brand] in the morning, there are oranges, there are lemons. Prepare a flavored drink. Prepare some Tupperwares with beans and egg and bring that [for your child] when you come to the consultation." Because they walk an hour and a half, two hours [to get here].

These words frame the indigenous people as irrational, irresponsible, ignorant, even lazy. They also reinforce and show a reliance on women as the primary transmitters of cultural knowledge (Bedford 2009). Ignoring structural barriers in the mothers' lives continues to contribute to a situation where indigenous women's mothering is problematic. These attitudes prove that the development offered by Oportunidades has limited cultural recognition, "while promoting economic policies that deepen indigenous structural poverty" (Bedford 2009:132). By ignoring the "disjuncture between globalizing discourses and localized social realities," the social suffering of the mothers (and their community) is likely to increase, thereby multiplying their losses and "contribut[ing] to the very suffering [the program seeks] to alleviate" (Whiteford and Manderson 2000:60).

The local consequences of Oportunidades are not perhaps evident in the immediate now, but they are likely to manifest themselves in the future, when the women have given up their local ideas of mothering in favor of the national model. They will have transformed their ideas of *Mexicano* motherhood to fall in line with *mestizo* motherhood—even though this change might not be entirely to their benefit or that of their children. The consequences of such a change affect more than simply the mothering practices of the women, impacting health, education, and future prospects for the children.

In rural villages, a diet of bread and lentils and processed meats and sodas is not necessarily better than corn, beans, chicken, and coffee, and an agricultural lifestyle is not necessarily worse than a low-paying job in a city. These are not hard and fast dichotomies. Indigenous people across Mexico—as with marginalized people across the world—are being squeezed at both ends. Most of these populations still have poor basic health—deficiency diseases, gastrointestinal issues, and tuberculosis—yet they are also increasingly susceptible to diseases of development—cancers, diabetes, and hypertension. Over the past seven years of my research, I have observed the consumption of junk food increase exponentially. The consumption of sodas in Mexico is already one of the highest in the world—accounting for over 20 percent of Pepsi's and 15 percent of Coca-Cola's worldwide sales (Leatherman and Goodman 2005). And while soda in Amatlán has historically been a luxury good and a symbol of great prestige, only consumed at feasts or important social functions, over the past few years, in the "coca-colonization" (Leatherman and Goodman 2005) of Mexico, it has taken on a more commonplace and daily role in people's diets. The reason for this change can be tied to the binge behavior (Wilk 2011) emerging from the increased cash flow of Oportunidades, where relative want alternates with relative abundance, leading to frenetic levels of consumption during the periods of abundance and to the multinational marketing efforts of Pepsi and Coca-Cola. The mothers will be held responsible for not taking care of their children's health and teeth, even though it is the cash from Oportunidades that enables this change in consumption in the first place. It is the very push for development—to be modern Mexicans with material prosperity—that underlies such competitive consumption.

The education that students receive in this region is mediocre at best. Though they are literate in a strict sense (on graduating, they receive a high school diploma), they are not given the literacy tools to become advocates and to have awareness of the larger societal problems: Paulo Freire's *concientizaçao*. David, one of the high school teachers who was originally trained as an accountant and decided to enter teaching in his middle years, felt that much of his teaching was a form of experimentation, as he was woefully underprepared to teach most topics.[4] Preferring to teach his own specialty, he had to admit, "But this is the system we have in indigenous schools, rural or otherwise." Students receive the right amount of education to work in semiskilled jobs, but not the kind of education that will produce productive middle-class citizens.

So where does the empowerment actually lie for these populations? The mothers are not empowered in a large political and social sense—the social engineering of Oportunidades effectively strips autonomy and self-worth. Their children—whose aspirations are directed away from the village—are often rudely awakened when their expectations meet reality. The mothers must then scramble to help their children regain their footing and achieve intended goals. When Lourdes—the strong and devoted *partera*—realized that her youngest son, Samuel, was unable to meet his goals of a university education, she confided that she considered moving to Mexico City to work as a maid so she could help him fund his dreams.

Deep structural factors underlie most race, class, and gender relations in Mexico. This is a nation riddled with overt and hidden *raciclasismo*. Self-conscious of its mixed indigenous and European identity, the population places much emphasis on phenotype as an indicator of social and economic background. Being in a lower class in Mexico often goes hand–in-hand with having indigenous ancestry—the greater indigenous ancestry one has, the lower one tends to be on the social ladder. Indigenous populations continue to live at the bottom of the economic scale—numbers show that 80 percent of indigenous people have high or very high levels of marginality, 64 percent of indigenous homes have piped water, 83.1 percent have electricity, while 43.7 percent have homes with earth floors. Additionally, in municipalities that have over 40 percent indigenous population, 56.8 percent of the population works in the primary sector and 30.7 percent receives no income for their labor. In Veracruz, 63.3 percent of the population over the age of fifteen is illiterate, while for indigenous people in general across the country, the percentage is 31.1 percent. Nationwide, 86.1 percent of the indigenous population has no access to health care (CDI 2009). Amatlán lies in the high marginality areas of the marginality maps created by the Comisión Nacional para el Desarrollo de los Pueblos Indígenas (CDI 2012). Indigenous women continue to be at a disadvantage to men nationwide regarding education and literacy, income, and poverty. Illiteracy rates for indigenous women nationwide is at 33.7 percent, compared to 19.1 percent for men. Rates for school in attendance for populations between six and twenty-three years old are 41.9 percent for women and 38.3 percent for men (Instituto Nacional de las Mujeres 2012). Urban feminization of poverty has also increased nationwide.

Because women are essentialized as caregivers by Oportunidades, they are made responsible for the health and educational well-being of their entire family. Cristina's words earlier, "It's just that as women we have to do everything," show the domestic burden borne by rural women. While a just-add-men-and-stir approach is not necessarily a solution, I would hope that men could be involved in certain aspects of Oportunidades—such as attending *pláticas* or taking the children to the health centers. This might encourage greater sharing of the duties surrounding childcare. I take to heart, however, Bedford's warning (2009:xxxi) that the current focus on empowered women living in a heterosexual, nuclear family arrangement with a loving and participative husband-father has been seen as a solution to "macroeconomic tensions." Though her intent is not to dismiss loving couplehood, she does offer important questions about gender role assumptions and the conventions of normality and equality are being used as the standard.

One of the main problems with Oportunidades is that it has morphed from its original design by economists and academics—as a stopgap measure that was to be the prologue for a broader structural change for poverty alleviation—to a program implemented and managed in a very different manner by politicians. In the process, it has lost its original intent and has become a political tool for vote capture. In turn, its fifteen years of touted success become expedient tools, and each government tries to own it in some way: The name change from Progresa to Oportunidades in 2000 (when the government changed from PRI to PAN) was not accidental. In renaming the program, the PAN has tried to own it and recapture people's votes in their favor.

Though I find much agency and strength among my friends in Amatlán, I am often disheartened about what the future will bring for them, and what new modernizing policies will be inflicted on them, as long as indigeneity continues to be seen in opposition to *mestizaje* and modernity. How can the country redress the legacies of *indigenismo* when so many of its welfare policies remain *indigenista?*

Cristina's suggestions for improving the program are probably the most grounded and straightforward. She said, "We should be well-treated. They should give us medications, because sometimes there are none [at the clinic]. And if there could be some place [at the clinic] where the patients can sit if it rains. [But mostly] more medications, better care." Though on the surface her suggestions are simple—infrastructure and a supply of medications—they also speak to the deeper issues all the women have echoed regarding their feeling of being mistreated and pushed aside. To provide someplace dry to protect from the rain the people one is trying to help is a simple courtesy that speaks volumes about dignity and human worth.

Niyahua—*I Am Leaving*

"She will get frightened when she sees all these monkeys." During a quick visit in early 2012 I took my toddler daughter to meet her many *abuelas* and *ahuis* in Amatlán.[5] Ofelia and Esperanza made this startling statement about how their faces would likely scare my daughter. Never before had I heard anyone in Amatlán utter such a self-disparaging, albeit semi-joking, comment about skin color and appearance. While everyone in the village was aware that they were indigenous and at the bottom of the economic and social pecking order, there was always a sense of dignity and of just going through the daily grind without thinking about oppressive forces of broader Mexico.

During the almost ten years I had been living and working in the region, I had observed an increase in people's sense of being the "other" and the "unwanted." While unable to attribute it directly to enrollment in Oportunidades and clinics, I do wonder at the compelling connection between people's identity and their participation in modernity. Pressure and derision from the media also complicates things. When all the variety shows have tall, buxom, thin women clearly of European descent dancing around in skimpy clothes, it is hard for indigenous women not to compare their petite, long-skirted selves to those images. A popular talent show watched every evening by most of the youth in the village had a truly dreadful skit where competitors were "taught" a *lengua indígena* (indigenous language). Using names from the Aztec pantheon, such as Huitzilopochtli or Tezcatlipoca, instead of modern-day Nahuatl, the show employed these words to mock the participants' appearance or abilities.[6] In a curious and no doubt unintentional twist to *indigenismo*, the impression this skit gave was that indigenous languages belonged only to a pre-Hispanic past—no living languages or people remained. The use of "fake" Nahuatl as an instrument for mockery undercut any dignity and pride held by modern-day indigenous populations.

In many ways, the story of Amatlán is the story of indigenous and marginalized people everywhere: every day they face poverty and disillusion with mainstream institutions and are told that they are not doing things right. I hope that the mothers' stories call attention to the racial and inequity issues in Mexico, especially regarding indigenous women. Still, they face their issues with humor and with a sense of strength. Women tactically envision their children's futures, scrambling to find ways to send them to university, their family's hopes and dreams riding on their shoulders.

Lourdes decided not to migrate to Mexico City, and soon after that, Samuel started his studies at the Universidad Veracruzana Intercultural— where his interest in communication led him to an exploration of the traditional dances of the region, which became the topic of his university thesis. He graduated with a *licenciatura* in 2012.[7] Cristina's eldest daughters graduated from high school, one of them obtaining a diploma in computing, prompting Cristina to dream of ways to set up a small Internet café in Amatlán. She was successful. Alicia and Estela continued to manage their large household, their needs often taking a backseat to the needs of their male relatives, their jobs and education. At the behest of her husband, Estela eventually moved to Mexico City with her two children, leaving her mother, Alicia, in charge of the household in Amatlán. Esperanza's role as a grandmother grew—as one of her daughters brought her own child for Esperanza to look after while she worked at the Kohler *maquiladora* (assembly plant) at one of the border towns. Camila moved to Mexico City after marriage and childbirth to live with her husband's sisters, while he worked as a policeman in northern Mexico; lack of money made her alternately consider getting a (dangerous) job as a policewoman or moving back to her husband's village—just a few miles from Amatlán. She chose the latter, deciding to bring up her young son in the familiarity of her own culture. Resiliently adjusting their lives to their changing circumstances, these mothers continue to manage their motherhood in the best way they can. They live their lives with dignity and humor—returning home with humor to deal with the indignities they face in the cities and hospitals, and with the patronizing *indigenismo*.

Notes

A Word on Nahuatl Pronunciation

1. Alan R. Sandstrom (1991) has a good set of notes on the pronunciation of Nahuatl in the region of Ixhuatlán. I have borrowed some of his suggestions here.

Introduction

1. All the names for the small villages are pseudonyms. I have used the real names for the larger towns and cities—Llano de Enmedio, Ixhuatlán de Madero, Álamo, and Poza Rica.
2. Bonfil Batalla (1996) proposed this idea in his analysis of the complex relationship among the various Mexicos.
3. Postectli (Pos-TEC-tlee) is part of a chain of seven hills, called Chikontepec (chee-CON-teh-pec) ("seven hills" in Nahuatl). They are very steep, conical hills protruding abruptly from the ground. The Postectli is the tallest hill (projecting more than six hundred meters straight up from the surrounding terrain) and the one most visible. It means "broken hill" in Nahuatl because a section at the top looks as though it broke off. Postectli is sacred to many of the indigenous groups of the area, not only the Nahua, and continues to receive yearly pilgrimages from all parts of the region. Gómez Martínez (2002) and Sandstrom (2003) provide in-depth descriptions of the various religious rituals and festivals centered on these hills.
4. *Telebachilleratos* (teh-leh-bah-chee-yeh-RAH-toes) are television-based high schools, which were established in Veracruz in 1980. The students receive a large part of their education through the state television program. This system has allowed more schools to be built in needy areas, which often suffer from teacher shortages. The television bridges this gap.

5. *Galeras* (gah-LEH-rahs) are tubular, metal-roofed, open structures used for special events.

6. *Zacahuil* (sah-cah-WHEEL) is an enormous *tamal* made from stone-ground maize mixed with various spices, wrapped tightly in banana leaves, and then baked in a clay oven. It is meat filled and can feed over twenty people. *Xamitl* (SHAH-mee-tl) is a sweet corn *tamal*. It is made only when sweet corn is available, before it ripens and is allowed to turn to maize.

7. *Mestizo* (meh-STEE-sow) originally meant a person of mixed indigenous and European descent; the term has come to include cultural mixture as well. See also Chapter 1, note 3 for a more in-depth explanation.

8. See Ruhl 2002 for an analysis of "willed" pregnancies.

9. Pentecostal missionaries first came into Amatlán in 1983 and introduced a new religious doctrine to the villagers. Though at first the conversion was slow (see Sandstrom 1991 for a very complete account of the conversion process to Pentecostalism in Amatlán), over the years more and more people converted to these beliefs to the extent that nowadays about 60 percent of the village is Pentecostal. The conversion of such a large number of people to Pentecostalism has had a major effect on the religious structure of the village. In the past, the entire village would organize religious events (such as Carnival or All Soul's Day) and everyone would participate. Nowadays, the few remaining Catholics consider many of these religious events to be too expensive for them to afford, and so they are not organized in such a fervent or elaborate manner as they used to be, with several of them going by the wayside.

10. Sandstrom (1975; 1978; 1998).

11. *Baja de matriz*, fallen uterus, is an ethnomedical category found across Latin America. The etiology is both physical (i.e., a fall, prolonged labor, or hot-cold differential) and social (i.e., lack of strength or lack of social support).

12. *Comadre* (f.) and *compadre* (m.) are terms for the adults in a parent-godparent relationship.

13. I took notes primarily by hand during these interviews, which were later transcribed with the help of research assistants. I also obtained supplementary data through the collection of over 150 plants used by the people as well as archival research and interviews with staff at the Ministry of Social Development (SEDESOL) and the National Population Council (CONAPO) in Mexico City.

14. Programa de Desarrollo Humano Oportunidades: the Opportunities Human Development Program. Oportunidades has been amply funded by the World Bank and the Inter-American Development Bank.

15. The program began under former president Ernesto Zedillo from the PRI party and was continued by his successor, Vicente Fox, who belonged to

the PAN. Originally named Progresa—an imperative form of "to progress"—it was renamed Oportunidades in 2002 by former president Vicente Fox's government.

16. Though Oportunidades is managed by SEDESOL, it is an interinstitu-
tional program that involves the Ministry of Public Education, the Ministry of Health, and the Mexican Institute for Social Insurance, as well as
state and municipal governments.

17. Slogans included "Let's become fewer" (*Hay que ser menos*); "The smaller
family is better off" (*La familia pequeña vive mejor*); "Ma'am, you decide if
you get pregnant" (*Señora, usted decide si se embaraza*); and "Family planning: It's a couple's choice" (*Planificación familiar: Es decisión de pareja*).

18. *Xinola* (she-NOH-lah) is a Nahuatl version of *señora* and refers to a married nonindigenous woman. (In Nahuatl, almost all Xs are pronounced
"SH.")

19. But as Robertson (2002:789) cautions, these identity categories often "ef-
face the complexity of [people's] personal and professional lives, not to men-
tion [their families'] histories." Indeed, for most of my first year in the field,
many people simply referred to me as "*la gringa*," lumping me in with the
collective "other" from abroad. My constant entreaties that I was not American, and that I was actually Mexican, fell on deaf ears. It was not until after
I had returned over and over that people realized that I straddled various
worlds, one of which was the indigenous world of Amatlán.

20. "*Ya no sirve.*"

21. Indeed, the most productive oil well in the world was found in this region
in the early twentieth century (Ruvalcaba Mercado, Pérez Zevallos, and
Herrera 2004).

22. *Ejidos* (eh-JEE-thos) are shared-use communal land established during the
Mexican agrarian reform in the early twentieth century. Though the system has been reformed many times, most notably during the administration of former president Carlos Salinas de Gortari in 1992, the Mexican
government continues to promote the use of communal land by a community.

23. *Corridos* (coh-RHEE-thos) are narrative songs or ballads of Mexico that
reflect some of the concerns and preoccupations of the population. They
were popularized during the Mexican revolution. A current form of *corridos* growing in popularity are *narcocorridos*—where the role of the drug
trade is discussed and often glorified.

24. A *comal* (coh-MAHL) is a smooth, flat, metal or earthenware griddle used
for cooking tortillas.

25. *Mole* is thick sauce with significant regional variations; in this region it is
made from dried chilies, onions, and tomatoes. It is usually served over
chicken, pork, or (during special events) turkey.

26. *Hija* (f.) and *hijo* (m.) are terms for "child" and are used to affectionately address a younger person; such address can also be considered slightly patronizing.

27. In 2010, when my own daughter was born and I called Esperanza to let her know, she happily exclaimed that she now had a *nieta* (granddaughter) and was extremely eager to meet her.

28. *Sobador(a)* (soh-bah-DOOR) is someone who uses massage or bonesetting in his or her healing practice.

29. *Solar* (soh-LAR) is the term used for the plot of land upon which the home is built, along with the surrounding home garden used for growing plants for construction, ornamentation, medicine, or food.

30. *Costumbre* (cohs-TOOM-breh) literally means "custom," but the terms is used throughout the Huasteca to refer to traditional religious and healing rituals that have strong connections to pre-Hispanic worldviews. A *curandero* (Spanish, healer) or a *tlamatiketl* (Nahuatl, person of knowledge) manages these rituals (see Sandstrom 1975, 1978, 1991, and 2003 for in-depth discussions of *costumbres* in Amatlán).

Chapter 1

1. A *hacienda* is a large, privately owned agrarian estate.

2. Don Eladio passed away in late 2011; he was well over one hundred years old.

3. *Mestizaje* originally meant a mixing of indigenous and European bloodlines. It was a biological process. The term has slowly changed meaning to include cultural mixture as well. So someone who eschews indigenous culture, yet is fully descended from indigenous blood, would be a *mestizo* by virtue of his or her behavior. Thus, when Mexico considers itself a *mestizo* nation, it actually refers to the cultural transformation of its population.

4. The government, aided by the media, was so successful at demonizing the Zapatistas that when in 2004 a group of Zapatistas forcibly evicted a wealthy land owner near Amatlán, the people of the village whispered with great concern about whether they would be next on this violent group's hit list.

5. A student of Franz Boas, Manuel Gamio is considered to be the father of Mexican anthropology. Following from Boas's historical particularism and concern with recording all details of vanishing groups, he emphasized what he termed "integral investigation," which emphasized a detailed study of a population integrated with its various social and natural environments through time (León-Portilla 1962).

6. In 1938, the Escuela Nacional de Antropología e Historia (ENAH) was created to further ideas of *indigenismo* in the governmental bureaucracy. Archaeologists and historians were important in recreating the past

through the most monumental findings, while cultural anthropologists were dedicated to "scientifically" integrating the indigenous population (Warman 1970).

7. Aguirre Beltrán (1991) defined "regions of refuge" as isolated areas (forests, deserts, mountains) where indigenous communities took refuge from mainstream political and economic pressures. Using a historical lens, he explains why indigenous communities are almost always found in highly marginalized and remote areas. These communities become satellites to the urban areas, and a very asymmetrically dependent relationship is created between them.

8. It should be noted that Lombardo emphasized the *respect* of indigenous leadership yet not their *political recognition*. This meant that the Mexican state was the ultimate political, economic, and legal authority.

9. The anthropologist Héctor Diaz-Polanco (1996) states that such a policy is very problematic because it emphasizes the nature of the indigenous population rather than the political condition or the abilities of the population to define the municipality, and in this way it segregates, corners, and encloses the indigenous population.

10. Former Mexican president Vicente Fox's government launched a major development and infrastructure project called the Plan Puebla Panamá, supported by the World Bank and the Inter-American Development Bank. This plan, renamed the Mesoamerica Project in 2008, has the goals of fostering economic development and increasing the richness of the human and natural capital of the Mesoamerican region. It is especially interested in "overcoming the enormous backwardness and inequality that severely hurts our country, and which are incompatible with the process of democratic consolidation" (Burch 2001, my translation). Dávila, Kessel, and Levy (the architect of Oportunidades) wrote an article proposing a major hydro-agronomal and transportational change to the south of Mexico. They state that the "southeast's social delay is, simultaneously, cause and effect of its productivity delay" (Dávila et al. 2002:210, my translation). As Burch (2001) points out, indigenous communities are seen as literal and figurative obstacles to this development.

11. The INI was officially dismantled in 2003.

12. This term arose over the media maelstrom that ensued after Enrique Peña Nieto, the presidential candidate for the PRI in the 2012 elections, made several public gaffes about the nature of the Mexican population. Within a space of a few short seconds, he twice repeated that what Mexico needed the most were "justice and *in*equality." In 2011, the blogger Geraldine Juárez referred to this slip-up as "accidental honesty" and coined the term *raciclasismo* to decry the elite classes' perception of the people they rule.

13. As the MDGs are a motivating justification for Oportunidades, it is worth noting that several analysts see the MDGs as distorting government

priorities. Brownbridge (2004) particularly critiques the use of large donors to fund projects, stating that this approach is doomed to fail as donors are volatile and unpredictable. He points out that most of the funding needs to be internally generated by the country in order to actually tackle poverty.

14. World Bank president Robert McNamara in 1979 first proposed the idea of conditionality.

15. Amartya Sen defined capabilities as the overall freedoms of people to lead the kind of lives they value—and have reason to value (1999:18).

16. Oportunidades requires one of the beneficiary women—the *promotora*—to locally manage the program and keep track of the beneficiaries; her purpose is to inform the women of the rules, meetings, and other conditions. She is elected by the beneficiary women in each village. A mirror position is the *auxiliar*, who is a liaison between the clinic and the women in each village.

17. By 2011 the amounts for the last year of high school were 840 pesos for boys and 960 pesos for girls (SEDESOL 2012a)

18. The rate of conversion at that time was one dollar to just over ten pesos, so this is approximately US$23.

19. The condition for students to receive this amount was for them to finish their last year of high school before the age of twenty-two.

20. Diaz-Cayeros et al. (2006) argue that support for the PAN (Partido Acción Nacional, National Action Party) among poor, urban Oportunidades beneficiaries was an integral component to Felipe Calderón's victory during the 2006 presidential election. Calderón was the successor of Vicente Fox, also from the PAN, and the president who pushed Oportunidades to its current scope and size.

21. PRI (Partido Revolucionario Institucional, Institutional Revolutionary Party) is the party that ruled Mexico for over seventy years after the Mexican Revolution. Its primary voting base was rural. Procampo (Pro-farm) is a subsidy for farmers, which provides farmers who grow staples (such as corn) with a fixed income payment per hectare (or hectare fraction) of farmland. Designed in 1993, it emerged as a way to subsidize and compensate national farmers for the "subsidies that their foreign competitors receive" (Apoyos y Servicios a la Comercializacion Agropecuaria [ASERCA] 2002).

22. Das et al. (2005) point out that *un*conditional cash would be used for other pressing necessities, not just the ones expected by the program.

23. Though not explicit in the directives about Oportunidades, state expansion is usually a significant part of the ideological framework of such a program—especially one that enrolls such a large proportion of the population.

24. The percentage of people living below the poverty line in Mexico in 2008 was 18.2 percent. This was based on a food-based definition of poverty.

Asset-based poverty was more than 47 percent (Central Intelligence Agency [CIA] 2012). Using various indicators—such as per capita income, average household educational delay, access to health services, access to social security, home construction/materials, access to basic services, access to food security, and degree of social cohesion—this rate is measured every few years. In Ixhuatlán de Madero, 84.7 percent of the population lived in poverty. For 99.6 percent of the municipality's population, at least one of the indicators listed above was lacking, while 81.5 percent lack at least three of these indicators (Consejo Nacional de Evaluación [CONEVAL] 2010).

25. *Pláticas* (PLAH-tee-cahs) are health, nutrition, and hygiene education sessions that mothers enrolled in Oportunidades must attend.

26. Agua Viva is an offshoot of Pentecostalism. As far as I could tell, it was brought in and maintained by missionaries from the United States.

27. *Chichi* (CHEE-chee) is the Nahuatl term for breast (and breastfeeding).

Chapter 2

1. Nancy Rose Hunt (1988:405) shows how in Africa, eugenicists linked the "degeneration of the races" to a concern with the centrality of imperial domination. Laura Briggs (2000) shows a similar concern with the political emancipation of white women in the United States, who were seen to be allowing the overly fertile darker-skinned populations to reproduce.

2. This trend is not unlike others across the globe, such as efforts to curb the risky behavior leading to STIs by using conditional cash transfers in Malawi.

3. Hunt (1988) discusses the use of puericulture among colonial powers in Belgian Congo in order to teach African mothers to reduce infant mortality. Puericulture was seen as a patriotic duty (for the Belgians, that is) in order to continue the production of black labor for the extractive economy dependent on their bodies.

4. Arranque Parejo en la Vida was created in 2003 to "provide information and quality health services to guarantee a healthy pregnancy, a safe birth, and a postpartum without complications to all Mexican women" (Secretaría de Salud 2002:29, my translation). It also seeks equality for development and growth for all children from birth until two years of age. Its primary aim is to decrease maternal and infant mortality by ensuring that a larger number of births occur in hospitals, by training traditional birth attendants and other medical personnel, and by improving medical infrastructures and facilities.

5. While baby slings were popularized in the US in the early twenty-first century, the only women who carried children in a *rebozo* in Mexico during the mid-twentieth century were indigenous or very poor.

6. Mexico City decriminalized abortion in 2007; women can receive an abortion up to the twelfth week of pregnancy. This policy is one of the most liberal for Latin America.

7. *Casa de salud* means "house of health," a simple clinic structure designed to promote community health. The one in Amatlán receives infrequent visits by the health-care professionals.

8. There is an increase of 11 to 14 percent in girls' enrollment in school in comparison with localities where there is no Oportunidades program.

9. Within this book I use two terms to describe midwives. The first is *partera* (the Mexican term for traditional midwife). The second is "traditional birth attendant" or its acronym, TBA.

10. Ofelia had an unexpected pregnancy in 2008, giving birth to a little girl. She thought she was no longer able to have children. Unfortunately, this pregnancy almost brought about the dissolution of her marriage. Her husband—who lived away most of the year due to his job as a policeman—was suspicious about her pregnancy, he was angry at the fact that he had another mouth to feed, and he did not accept the child as his own. In 2009, Ofelia was still trying to put the fragments of her once very strong marriage back together, while taking care of her children and home.

11. Various references to Catholic saints related to pregnancy and birth exist: San Ramón Nonato, Saint Brigid, and the Virgin of Guadalupe.

12. Pitocin, the hormone that is used medically during birth, mimics oxytocin by contracting the uterus and encouraging contractions and pushing. It is used to speed up the birth. These contractions are usually much stronger than the ones occurring through the body's production of oxytocin, so the women's comments that they made the birth more comfortable in fact contradict what is usually known about this hormone. Perhaps for these women, the shorter labor meant it was more comfortable, as there was less time of discomfort.

13. *Tentsocopale* (tent-sow-coh-PAH-leh) is the local term for what seems to be newborn tetanus, which claimed the lives of many infants before medical care arrived in the area.

14. This hospital model—which integrates biomedical and indigenous forms of medicine—is rare in Mexico. Cuetzalan is often held up as a classic example of this integration. However, the actual "integration" is questionable—each medical system is relegated to a separate building. Additionally, the indigenous practitioners receive professionalization by clinicians, but clinicians are not in turn professionalized to understand local forms of healing.

Chapter 3

1. Chapter I, Article 4 of the Mexican Constitution states, "Every person has the right to decide, in a free, responsible, and informed manner, the number and spacing of his or her children."

2. This program has had various maxims over the years, including "*la familia pequeña vive mejor*" (a small family is better off) and "*pocos hijos para darles mucho*" (few children to give them a lot).

3. Chicontepec is often referred to colloquially as Chicón.

4. In response to a historical hierarchical access to health care, Mexico reformed its General Health Law in 2003 to create a system to guarantee that marginalized populations received financial support for health care. This new system was named Seguro Popular (People's Health Insurance) (Knaul et al. 2007). All the government-run clinics and hospitals across the country accept Seguro Popular.

5. *Mija* is a contraction of *mi hija*—my child. It is used as a slightly patronizing form of address to those of lower class or of younger age than one's self. See also Introduction, note 26.

6. PRD is the Partido de la Revolución Democrática, the Party of the Democratic Revolution.

7. This description of the politics of health care in Mexico was provided to me by Mr. Christopher J. F. Smith, a businessman and longtime resident of Mexico.

8. This authority is intended, yet not openly articulated, in planning documents and official justifications of the program.

9. *Las tenemos bien amarraditas.*

Chapter 4

1. *La gente ha ido despertando.* This is usually used to suggest that people are more aware and awake about the larger world.

2. All of these are brands of powdered milk, calcium drinks, or chocolate milk drinks.

3. *Tostes* are spicy fried and salted commercially made wheat chips.

4. *Milpa* (MEEL-pah) is agricultural land used for the production of food crops; in Amatlán it usually refers to cornfields.

5. *Petates* (peh-TAH-teh) are woven straw mats that people sleep on. In Nahuatl it is *petlatl.*

6. *Chamacos* (chah-MAH-cos) is a Mexican word for kids.

7. Dulce's eldest son was about eleven in 2007. He is also perceived to be *trastornado* by the villagers, as he frequently behaves inappropriately (going about naked, for instance) and has some other sorts of developmental and cognitive issues.

8. *Pilón* (pea-LON) is raw, unprocessed sugar from sugar cane. The cane juice is cooked and reduced until it forms thick brown liquid. It is then poured into hollowed-out molds made from cane stalks cut to about 30 cm length; they are allowed to harden. The round bricks of *pilón* are used to sweeten any food product made by the people, from coffee, to juice drinks, to bread.

9. This is particularly true for middle-class women who do not work outside of the home.
10. The doctor referred to the women as *marginadas*—the marginalized.

Chapter 5

1. The new term for *promotora*.
2. Doctor Braulio was actually very patient with the women as well as particularly polite. While it is common to find that physicians and others in authority address indigenous and low-income women as "*tu*" (informal form of "you"), Doctor Braulio always addressed them as *doña* (akin to "ma'am") and used "*usted*" (formal "you").
3. Sotero narrated various long stories about the various ways that Conejo tricked Coyote. In one story, Conejo convinced Coyote to take his place in a sack, causing Coyote to be beaten by an old lady for eating her *frijoles* (beans). Conejo then convinced Coyote that if he did not hold up a heavy boulder, the world would end. Conejo told Coyote he would go in search of food while Coyote held up the boulder, but he never returned. Later, Coyote was increasingly hungry and angrily said, "That Conejo has really tricked me. When I next see him I will definitely eat him." Sotero continued, "So he searched and searched and found him on the water's edge and said, 'Now I will definitely eat you Conejo' he said. 'You have tricked me too much' he said. 'I will now eat you' he said. 'There is a lot to eat' said Conejo. 'Cheese, [or] whatever you want.' Because Conejo was holding a piece of cheese and the Coyote wanted to eat it, because it is delicious. 'And where did you get that from?' 'It is there,' says Conejo [pointing]. It was the moon reflected in the water. It was the moon. 'And how do you get it out of there?' 'I tie a stone around my neck' he says." Sotero laughed and so did his listeners. He continued, "'I tie a stone around my neck and I jump in. And then I get the cheese out.' And that is what Coyote did. But he did not get anything. He almost drowned! It took a lot of effort to get out of that one. And when he came out he said, 'Whenever I find that Conejo I have to eat him,' he said." Coyote's travails ended when Conejo finally outwitted him by tricking him into a barrel filled with fireworks—which Conejo lit on fire. Sotero ended with a laugh: "There the Coyote was burned. Conejo bested him. Coyote did not eat him."
4. *Culto* (COOL-toh) is used both for Pentecostal worship and for the actual religious group; that is, people belong to the *culto*, and they practice *culto*.
5. Perhaps equally significant in Esperanza's story is the use of politics in this region and its connection to health. While she lauds Doctor Gastón for helping to treat her son from his own medicine cabinet, the story she tells about his sliding fee scale based on political support shows him to be as much of a political animal and opportunist as Doctor Fermín. Physicians

in the region have much status and often use this status and position for political purposes—gaining power and wealth that can potentially negatively damage the low-income populations of the region.

Conclusion

1. The UVI (it is pronounced as the acronym OOH-vee) is a recently established university system in Veracruz, which began statewide in 2004 with the goal of creating a cross-cultural and hybrid education that acknowledges the polysemous knowledge of the indigenous communities at which it is aimed. All students enroll in the primary major of intercultural development management while concentrating on any of the following subbranches: communication, sustainability, languages, rights/laws, and health. Ávila Pardo and Mateos Cortés (2008:80) point out that this educational system eschews the Eurocentric, logocentric, and urban educational system and aims to reorient the idea of a university to integrate social consciousness by creating spaces to incorporate knowledge that is usually disdained in mainstream higher education.

2. *Nopales* (noh-PAH-lehs) are the paddles or leaves of the prickly pear cactus. They belong to the family Cactaceae. They are eaten in large quantities across Mexico; their texture is both crisp like a green bean but also mucilaginous. They are nutritious and medicinally effective, especially for diabetes and high blood pressure.

3. *Chayotes* (cha-YOH-tehs) are an edible fruit belonging to the gourd family, Cucurbitaceae. This is the same family as cucumbers, melons, and squash.

4. I met David when he heard from Samuel and Jacqueline that I was teaching English. Both of them were his students at the high school. He decided to join my small group of students. The irony that one of the subjects he taught at school was English was not lost on us.

5. *Abuelas* is Spanish for "grandmothers," and *ahuis* (AH-wee), Nahuatl for "aunts" (fictive kin, usually).

6. Huitzilopochtli (we-tsee-loh-POSH-tlee) was the patron god of the Aztecs (Mexicas) of Tenochtitlan, often associated with war, sacrifice, and the sun. Tezcatlipoca (tes-cah-tlee-POH-cah) was also a central god to the Aztecs, associated with many things, including the night sky, discord, beauty, and obsidian.

7. A *licenciatura* is comparable to a bachelor of arts degree.

References

Abu-Lughod, Lila
    1990   The Romance of Resistance: Tracing Transformations of Power through Bedouin Women. American Ethnologist 17(1):41–55.

Adato, Michelle
    2008   Integrating Survey and Ethnographic Methods to Evaluate Conditional Cash Transfer Programs. Report. Washington, DC: International Food Policy Research Institute.

Adato, Michelle, and John Hoddinott
    2007   Conditional Cash Transfer Programs: A "Magic Bullet" for Reducing Poverty? 2020 Focus Brief on the World's Poor and Hungry People. Report. Washington, DC: International Food Policy Research Institute.

Administration for Children and Families (ACF)
    2012   The Healthy Marriage Initiative. U.S. Department of Health and Human Services. *acf.gov/healthymarriage/about/mission. html#notabout*. Accessed August 3, 2012.

Aguirre Beltrán, Gonzalo
    1991[1967] Regiones de Refugio. México, DF: Instituto Indigenista Interamericano INI.

Ahearn, Laura
    2001   Language and Agency. Annual Review of Anthropology 30:109–37.

Alarcón-Gonzáles, Diana, and Terry McKinley
    1999   The Adverse Effects of Structural Adjustment on Working Women in Mexico. Latin American Perspectives 23(3):103–17.

Allen, Denise R.
    2002   Managing Motherhood, Managing Risk: Fertility and Danger in West Central Tanzania. Ann Arbor: University of Michigan Press.

Allison, Anne
    1996   Permitted and Prohibited Desires: Mothers, Comics, and Censorship in Japan. Boulder: Westview.

Anderson, Benedict.
    1991   Imagined Communities: Reflections on the Spread and Origin of
            Nationalism. London: Verso.

Apoyos y Servicios a la Comercializacion Agropecuaria (ASERCA)
    2002   Objetivo. *www.aserca.gob.mx/artman/publish/article_183.asp*.
            Accessed April 19, 2011.

Appadurai, Arjun
    1996   Modernity at Large: Cultural Dimensions of Globalization.
            Minneapolis: University of Minnesota Press.

Appell, Annette R.
    1998   On Fixing "Bad" Mothers and Saving Their Children. *In* "Bad"
            Mothers: The Politics of Blame in Twentieth-Century America. Molly
            Ladd-Taylor and Lauri Umansky, eds. Pp. 356–80. New York: New
            York University Press.

Ariel de Vidas, Anath
    2005   La Bella Durmiente: El Norte de Veracruz. Nuevo Mundo Mundos
            Nuevos. *nuevomundo.revues.org/574*. Accessed September 23, 2010.

Arizpe, Lourdes
    1993   Cultura y Cambio Global: Percepciones Sociales Sobre
            la Deforestación en la Selva Lacandona. México, DF: Editor
            Miguel Ángel Porrúa.

Ávila Pardo, Adriana, and Laura S. Mateos Cortés
    2008   Configuración de Actores y Discursos Híbridos en la Creación de la
            Universidad Veracruzana Intercultural. Travaux et recherches dans
            les Amériques du Centre 53:64–82.

Azuela, Mariano
    2008[1916] Los de Abajo. New York: Penguin Classics.

Baird, Sarah, Ephraim Chirwa, Craig McIntish, and Berk Özler
    2009   The Short-Term Impacts of a Schooling Conditional Cash Transfer
            Program on the Sexual Behavior of Young Women. Impact Evaluation
            Series: Policy Research Working Paper 5089. Washington, DC: World
            Bank.

Barlow, Kathleen
    2004   Critiquing the "Good Enough" Mother: A Perspective Based on the
            Murik of Papua New Guinea. Ethos 32(4):514–37.

Bartolomé, Miguel, and Alicia Barabas
    1999   Configuraciones Étnicas en Oaxaca: Perspectivas Etnográficas Para
            las Autonomías. México, DF: Instituto Nacional de Antropología
            e Historia/Instituto Nacional Indigenista/Consejo Nacional para la
            Cultura y las Artes.

Bassin, Donna, Margaret Honey, and Meryle M. Kaplan
  1994   Introduction. *In* Representations of Motherhood. Donna Bassin,
          Margaret Honey, and Meryle M. Kaplan, eds. Pp. 1–28. New
          Haven: Yale University Press.

Basso, Keith
  1979   Portraits of the White Man: Linguistic Play and Cultural Symbols
          among the Western Apache. Cambridge: Cambridge University
          Press.

Basu, Alaka M.
  2002   Why Does Education Lead to Lower Fertility? A Critical Review of
          Some of the Possibilities. World Development 30(10):1779–90.

Bedford, Kate
  2006   The Imperative of Male Inclusion: How Institutional Context
          Influences World Bank Gender Policy. International Feminist
          Journal of Politics 9(3):289–311.
  2009   Developing Partnerships: Gender, Sexuality, and the Reformed
          World Bank. Minneapolis: University of Minnesota Press.

Berger, Jeffery T., Jack Coulehan, and Catherine Belling
  2004   Humor in the Physician-Patient Encounter. Archive of Internal
          Medicine 164(8):825–30.

Billings, Deborah L, Claudia Moreno, Celia Ramos, Deyanira González de León,
Ruben Ramírez, Leticia Villaseñor Martínez, and Mauricio Rivera Díaz
  2002   Constructing Access to Legal Abortion Services in Mexico City.
          Reproductive Health Matters 10(19):86–94.

Bliss, Katherine
  2002   Compromised Positions: Prostitution, Public Health, and Gender
          Politics in Revolutionary Mexico City. University Park: Penn State
          University Press.

Blumberg, Rae L.
  1988   Income under Female versus Male Control: Hypotheses from a
          Theory of Gender Stratification and Data from the Third World.
          Journal of Family Issues 9(1):51–84.

Boddy, Patricia
  2007   Civilizing Women: British Crusades in Colonial Sudan. Princeton:
          Princeton University Press.

Bonfil Batalla, Guillermo
  1996   México Profundo: Reclaiming a Civilization. Philip Dennis, trans.
          Austin: University of Texas Press.

Borghi, Jo, Apamaa Somanathan, Craig Lissner, and Anne Mills
   2006   Mobilising Financial Resources for Maternal Health. Lancet
           368:1457–65.

Bourdieu, Pierre
   1977   Outline of a Theory of Practice. Cambridge: Cambridge University
           Press

Bourgois, Philippe, and Jeff Schonberg
   2007   Intimate Apartheid: Ethnic Dimensions of Habitus among
           Homeless Heroin Injectors. Ethnography 8(1):7–32.

Brading, David A.
   1988   Manuel Gamio and Official Indigenismo in Mexico. Bulletin of
           Latin American Research 7(1):75–89.

Braff, Lara
   2008   Fertility Care and "Overpopulation": Imagining Mexico's Social
           Body. Paper presented at the 68th Annual Meeting of the Society for
           Applied Anthropology, Memphis, TN, March 27, 2008.
   2009   Assisted Reproduction and Population Politics: Creating "Modern"
           Families in Mexico City. Anthropology News 50(2):5–6.

Bridges, Khiara
   2007   Wily Patients, Welfare Queens, and the Reiteration of Race. The
           Texas Journal of Women and the Law 17(1):1–66.

Briggs, Laura
   2000   The Race of Hysteria: "Overcivilization" and the "Savage" Woman
           in Late Nineteenth-Century Obstetrics and Gynecology. American
           Quarterly 52(2):246–73.

Brownbridge, Martin
   2004   Financing the Millennium Development Goals: Is More Public
           Spending the Best Way to Meet Poverty Reduction Targets. Health
           Policy and Development 2(1):40–47.

Browner, Carole H.
   2000   Situating Women's Reproductive Activities. American
           Anthropologist 102(4):773–88.

Browner, Carole H., and Joanne Leslie
   1995   Women, Work, and Household Health in the Context of
           Development. In Gender and Health: An International Perspective.
           Carolyn F. Sargent and Caroline B. Brettell, eds. Pp. 242–59. Upper
           Saddle River: Prentice-Hall.

Browner, Carole H., and Carolyn Sargent
2011   Introduction. *In* Reproduction, Globalization, and the State: New
        Theoretical and Ethnographic Perspectives. Carole Browner and
        Carolyn Sargent, eds. Pp. 1–18. Durham: Duke University Press.

Burch, Sally
2001   El Istmo Mesoamericano: Globalización, Ecología y Seguridad.
        CIMAC Noticias. *www.cimacnoticias.com.mx/site/index.*
        php?id=29449&print=1&no_cache=1. Accessed March 15, 2009.

Cabrera, Gustavo
1994   Demographic Dynamics and Development: The Role of Population
        Policy in Mexico. Supplement, "The New Politics of Population:
        Conflict and Consensus in Family Planning," Population and
        Development Review 20:105–20.

Campos-Navarro, Roberto
2010   La Enseñanza de la Antropología Médica y la Salud Intercultural
        en México: Del Indigenismo Culturalista del Siglo XX a la
        Interculturalidad en Salud del Siglo XXI. Revista Peruana de
        Medicina Experimental y Salud Pública 27(1):114–22.

Cartwright, Sheree
2008   The Shifting Paid Work and Family Life Experiences and Cultural
        Habitus of Motherhood. International Journal of the Humanities
        5(12):139–49.

Castro, Arachu
2004   Contracepting at Childbirth: The Integration of Reproductive Health
        and Population Policies in Mexico. *In* Unhealthy Health Policy: A
        Critical Anthropological Examination. Arachu Castro and Merrill
        Singer, eds. Pp. 133–44. Walnut Creek, CA: Altamira.

Castro, Arachu, and Merrill Singer
2004   Introduction: Anthropology and Health Policy: A Critical
        Perspective. *In* Unhealthy Health Policy. Arachu Castro and Merrill
        Singer, eds. Pp. xi–xx. Walnut Creek, CA: Altamira.

Central Intelligence Agency (CIA)
2012   Mexico. CIA World Factbook. *https://www.cia.gov/library/*
        publications/the-world-factbook/geos/mx.html. Accessed April 23,
        2012.

Chavez, Leo
2004   A Glass Half Empty: Latina Reproduction and Public Discourse.
        Human Organization 63(2):173–88.

Chen, Junjie
    2011   Globalizing, Reproducing, and Civilizing Rural Subjects: Population
            Control Policy and Constructions of Rural Identity in China. *In*
            Reproduction, Globalization, and the State: New Theoretical and
            Ethnographic Perspectives. Carole Browner and Carolyn Sargent, eds.
            Pp. 38–52. Durham: Duke University Press.

Clark, Lauren
    1993   Gender and Generation in Poor Women's Household Health
            Production Experiences. Medical Anthropology Quarterly
            7(4):386–402.

Clifton, James
    1990   The Invented Indian: Cultural Fictions and Government Policies.
            New Brunswick: Transaction.

Colen, Shellee
    1995   "Like a Mother to Them": Stratified Reproduction and West Indian
            Childcare Workers and Employers in New York. *In* Conceiving the New
            World Order: The Global Politics of Reproduction. Faye Ginsburg and
            Rayna Rapp, eds. Pp. 78–102. Berkeley: University of California Press.

Collins, Patricia H.
    1994   Shifting the Center. *In* Representations of Motherhood. Donna
            Bassin, Margaret Honey, and Meryle M. Kaplan, eds. Pp. 56–74. New
            Haven: Yale University Press.

Comisión Nacional para El Desarrollo de los Pueblos Indígenas (CDI)
    2008a   Antecedentes. Ley de Creación del Instituto Nacional Indigenista. *www.
            cdi.gob.mx/index.php?option=com_content&task=view&id=3&Itemid=6.*
            Accessed March 15, 2012.
    2008b   Texto Vigente. Ley de Creación del Instituto Nacional Indigenista.
            *www.cdi.gob.mx/index.php?option=com_content&view=article&id=5&
            Itemid=8.* Accessed March 15, 2012.
    2009   Indicadores Socioeconómicos de los Pueblos Indígenas de México,
            2002. *www.cdi.gob.mx/index.php?option=com_content&
            task=view&id=206&Itemid=49.* Accessed January 12, 2011.
    2012   Municipios con 40% y Más de Población Indígena, Según Grado de
            Marginación, México, 2000. *www.cdi.gob.mx/indicadores/mapa04.html.*
            Accessed April 15, 2012.

Consejo Nacional de Evaluación de la Politica de Desarrollo Social (CONEVAL)
    2010   Medición de la Pobreza en México 2010, a Escala Municipal. *www.
            coneval.gob.mx/cmsconeval/rw/pages/medicion/multidimencional/
            informacion_municipios.es.do.* Accessed April 23, 2011.

Consejo Nacional de Población (CONAPO)
    2004   Carpeta Informativa: 11 de Julio, Día Mundial de Población.
            México, DF: Consejo Nacional de Población.
    2012   Indicadores Demográficos Básicos. *www.conapo.gob.mx/*
            en/CONAPO/Indicadores_demograficos_basicos. Accessed August 3,
            2012.

Cornwall, Andrea, and Karen Brock
    2005   What Do Buzzwords Do for Development Policy? A Critical Look
            at "Participation," "Empowerment," and "Poverty Reduction." Third
            World Quarterly 26(7):1043–60.

Coser, Rose L.
    1959   Some Social Functions of Laughter: A Study of Humor in a Hospital
            Setting. Human Relations 12:171–82.

Cosminsky, Sheila
    2001   Midwifery across Generations: A Modernizing Midwife in
            Guatemala. Medical Anthropology 20(4):345–78.

Craven, Christa
    2005   Claiming Respectable American Motherhood: Homebirth Mothers,
            Medical Officials, and the State. Medical Anthropology Quarterly
            19(2):194–215.

Davies, Christie
    1990   Ethnic Humor around the World. Bloomington: Indiana University
            Press.

Das, Jishnu, Quy-Toan Do, and Berk Özler
    2005   Reassessing Conditional Cash Transfer Programs. The World Bank
            Research Observer 20(1):57–80.

Dávila, Enrique, Georgina Kessel, and Santiago Levy
    2002   El Sur También Existe: Un Ensayo sobre el Desarrollo Regional de
            México. Economía Mexicana Nueva Época 11(2):205–61.

De la Peña, Guillermo
    1995   La Ciudad Étnica en el México Contemporáneo. Multiculturalismo
            6:116–40.

Diario Oficial
    2002   Diario Oficial de la Federación. *dof.gob.mx.* Accessed April 16, 2011.

Díaz-Cayeros, Alberto, Federico Estévez, and Beatriz Magaloni
    2006   Buying-Off the Poor: Effects of Targeted Benefits in the 2006
            Presidential Race. Paper presented at the Conference on the Mexico
            2006 Panel Study, Boston. November 30–December 2, 2006.

Díaz-Polanco, Héctor
  1996   Autonomía Regional: La Autonomía de los Pueblos Indios. México,
          DF: Siglo XXI Editores.

Dore, Elizabeth
  2000   One Step Forward, Two Steps Back: Gender and the State in
          Latin America's Long Nineteenth Century. *In* Hidden Histories of
          Gender and the State in Latin America. Elizabeth Dore and Maxine
          Molyneux, eds. Pp. 3–32. Durham: Duke University Press.

Douglas, Mary
  1986   How Institutions Think. Syracuse: Syracuse University Press.

Downe, Pamela J.
  1999   Laughing When It Hurts: Humor and Violence in the Lives of
          Costa Rican Prostitutes. Women's Studies International Forum
          22(1):63–78.

Dudgeon, Matthew
  2012   Conceiving Risk in K'iche' Maya Reproduction. *In* Risk,
          Reproduction, and Narratives of Experience. Lauren Fordyce and
          Aminata Maraesa, eds. Pp.17–36. Nashville: Vanderbilt University
          Press.

Escobar, Arturo
  1995   Encountering Development: The Making and Unmaking of the
          Third World. Princeton: Princeton University Press.

Escobar Ohmstede, Antonio
  1998   Historia de los Pueblos Indígenas de México: De la Costa a la Sierra,
          las Huastecas, 1750–1900. México, DF: CIESAS-INI.

Esposito, Robert
  2008   Bíos: Biopolitics and Philosophy. Timothy Campbell,
          trans. Minneapolis: University of Minnesota Press.

Ewald, François
  1986   Bio-Power. History of the Present 2:8–9.

Farmer, Paul
  2006   Foreword: Unraveling Fertility and Power. *In* Reproducing
          Inequities: Poverty and the Politics of Population in Haiti. By
          M. Catherine Maternowska. Pp. ix–xv. New Brunswick: Rutgers
          University Press.

Fordyce, Lauren
  2008   Birthing the Diaspora: Technologies of Risk among Haitians in
          South Florida. Ph.D. dissertation, Department of Anthropology,
          University of Florida.

2012   Imaging Maternal Responsibility: Prenatal Diagnosis and Ultrasound among Haitians in South Florida. *In* Risk, Reproduction, and Narratives of Experience. Lauren Fordyce and Aminata Maraesa, eds. Pp. 191–209. Nashville: Vanderbilt University Press.

Foucault, Michel
1991   Governmentality. *In* The Foucault Effect: Studies in Governmentality. Graham Burchell, Colin Gordon, and Peter Miller, eds. Pp. 87–104. Chicago: University of Chicago Press.
1995[1977] Discipline and Punish. A. M. Sheridan Smith, trans. New York: Vintage.

Fraser, Gertrude
1995   Modern Bodies, Modern Minds: Midwifery and Reproductive Change in an African-American Community. *In* Conceiving the New World Order: The Global Politics of Reproduction. Faye D. Ginsburg and Rayna Rapp, eds. Pp. 42–58. Berkeley: University of California Press.

Freud, Sigmund
2003[1905] The Joke and Its Relation to the Subconscious. New York: Penguin Classics.

Freyermuth, Graciela, and Paola Sesia
2006   Del Curanderismo a la Influenza Aviaria: Viejas y Nuevas Perspectivas de la Antropología Médica. Desacatos 20:9–28.

Fujita, Mariko
1989   It's All the Mother's Fault: Childcare and the Socialization of Working Mothers in Japan. Journal of Japanese Studies 15(1):67–91.

Gamio, Manuel
2010[1916] Forjando Patria: Pro Nacionalismo. Fernando Armstrong-Fumero, trans. Boulder: University of Colorado Press.

Gardner, Katy, and David Lewis
2005   Beyond Development? *In* The Anthropology of Development and Globalization: From Classical Political Economy to Contemporary Neoliberalism. Marc Edelman and Angelique Haugerud, eds. Pp. 352–59. Malden, MA: Blackwell.

Gellner, Ernesto
1983   Nations and Nationalism. Ithaca: Cornell University Press.

Ghose, Malini
  2001   Women and Empowerment through Literacy. *In* The Making of
          Literate Societies. David R. Olson and Nancy Torrance, eds. Pp.
          296–316. Oxford: Blackwell.

Ginsburg, Faye D., and Rayna Rapp
  1991   The Politics of Reproduction. Annual Review of Anthropology
          20:311–43.
  1995   Introduction. *In* Conceiving the New World Order: The Global
          Politics of Reproduction. Faye D. Ginsburg and Rayna Rapp, eds.
          Pp. 1–18. Berkeley: University of California Press.

Goldade, Kate
  2007   "Health Is Hard Here" or "Health for All"? The Politics of Blame,
          Gender, and Healthcare for Undocumented Migrants in Costa
          Rica. Paper presented at the Annual Meeting of the American
          Anthropological Association, Washington, DC, November 28–
          December 2, 2007.

Goldstein, Donna M.
  2003   Laughter out of Place: Race, Class, Violence, and Sexuality in a
          Rio Shantytown. Berkley: University of California Press.

Gómez Martínez, Arturo
  2002   Tlaneltokilli: La Espiritualidad de los Nahuas Chicontepecanos.
          México: Ediciones del Programa de Desarrollo Cultural de la
          Huasteca.

González, Roberto J.
  2004   From Indigenismo to Zapatismo: Theory and Practice in Mexican
          Anthropology. Human Organization 63(2):141–50.

González Montes, Soledad
  2008   Violencia Contra las Mujeres, Derechos, y Ciudadanía en Contextos
          Rurales e Indígenas de México. Convergencia 16(50):165–85.

Gramsci, Antonio
  1978   Quaderni del Carcere: Selections from the Prison Notebooks of
          Antonio Gramsci. Quintin Hoare and Geoffrey Nowell Smith, eds.
          and trans. New York: International.

Greenhalgh, Susan
  2005   Globalization and Population Governance in China. *In* Global
          Assemblages: Technology, Politics, and Ethics as Anthropological
          Problems. Aihwa Ong and Stephen J. Collier, eds. Pp. 354–72.
          Oxford: Blackwell.

Gutmann, Matthew
  2011   Planning Men out of Family Planning: A Case Study from Mexico.
          In Reproduction, Globalization, and the State: New Theoretical and

Ethnographic Perspectives. Carole Browner and Carolyn Sargent, eds. Pp. 53–67. Durham: Duke University Press.

Hacking, Ian
1991   How Should We Do the History of Statistics? *In* The Foucault Effect: Studies in Governmentality. Graham Burchell, Colin Gordon, and Peter Miller, eds. Pp. 181–95. Chicago: University of Chicago Press.

Harker, Richard K.
1984   On Reproduction, Habitus, and Education. British Journal of Sociology of Education 5(2):117–27.

Hart, Marjolein 't
2007   Humour and Social Protest: An Introduction. Internationaal Instituut voor Sociale Geschiedenis 52:1–20.

Hechter, Michael
1999   Internal Colonialism: The Celtic Fringe in British National Development. New Brunswick: Transaction.

Hernández Bautista, Paulino, Herminio Farías Bautista,
Pedro Silvestre Zavala, and José Barón Larios
2004   Chicomexóchitl: La Leyenda del Maíz. *In* La Huasteca, un Recorrido por Su Diversidad. Jesús Ruvalcaba Mercado, Juan Manuel Pérez Zevallos, and Octavio Herrera, ed. Pp. 369–78. México, DF: CIESAS.

Hernández Castillo, Rosalva A.
2001   La Otra Frontera: Identidades Múltiples en el Chiapas Poscolonial. México, DF: CIESAS.

Hill, Jane H., and Kenneth C. Hill
1986   Speaking Mexicano: Dynamics of Syncretic Language in Central Mexico. Tucson: University of Arizona Press.

Hong, Nathaniel
2010   Mow 'Em All Down Grandma: The "Weapon" of Humor in Two Danish World War II Occupation Scrapbooks. International Journal of Humor Research 23(1):27–64.

Huber, Brad, and Alan Sandstrom, eds.
2001   Mesoamerican Healers. Austin: University of Texas Press

Hunt, Nancy Rose
1988   "Le bébé en brousse": European Women, African Birth Spacing, and Colonial Intervention in Breast Feeding in the Belgian Congo. International Journal of African Historical Studies 21(3):401–32.
1990   Domesticity and Colonialism in Belgian Africa: Usumbura's Foyer Social, 1946–1960. Signs 15(3):447–74.

Instituto Mexicano del Seguro Social (IMSS)
    2012   Padrón de Beneficiarios, Instituto Mexicano Del Seguro Social
             Unidad IMSS-Oportunidades. División de Información IMSS
             Oportunidades. *www.imss.gob.mx/programas/oportunidades/Pages/
             inf_est.aspx.* Accessed August 6, 2012.

Instituto Nacional de las Mujeres (INMUJER)
    2012   Indicadores Básicos. *estadistica.inmujeres.gob.mx/formas/panorama_
             general.php?menu1=7&IDTema=7&pag=1.* Accessed April 23, 2012.

Instituto Nacional para el Federalismo y el Desarrollo Municipal (INAFED)
    2011   Enciclopedia de los Municipios de México: Estado de Veracruz de
             Ignacio de la Llave. *www.e-local.gob.mx/work/templates/enciclo/vera-
             cruz.* Accessed July 20, 2011.

Inter-American Development Bank (IDB)
    2003   Evaluation as a Tool. Ideas for Development in the Americas 1:5.

Ivry, Tsipy
    2007   Embodied Responsibility: Pregnancy in the Eyes of Japanese
             Ob-Gyns. Sociology of Health and Illness 29(2):251–74.

Jeffery, Roger, and Alaka M. Basu, eds.
    1996   Girls' Schooling, Women's Autonomy, and Fertility Change in South
             Asia. New Delhi: Sage.

Jenkins, Gwynne
    2003   Burning Bridges: Policy, Practice, and the Destruction of Midwifery
             in Rural Costa Rica. Social Science and Medicine 56:1893–909.

Johnson, Paige
    2002   The Use of Humor and Its Influences on Spirituality and Coping in
             Breast Cancer Survivors. Oncology Nursing Forum 29(4):691–95.

Jolly, Margaret
    1998   Introduction. *In* Maternities and Modernities: Colonial and
             Postcolonial Experiences in Asia and the Pacific. Kalpana Ram and
             Margaret Jolly, eds. Pp. 1–25. Cambridge: Cambridge University
             Press.

Jordan, Brigitte
    1993   Birth in Four Cultures: A Cross-Cultural Investigation of Childbirth
             in Yucatán, Holland, Sweden, and the United States. Prospect
             Heights, IL: Waveland.
    1997   Authoritative Knowledge and Its Construction. *In* Childbirth and
             Authoritative Knowledge: Cross-Cultural Perspectives. Robbie E. Davis-
             Floyd and Carolyn F. Sargent, eds. Pp. 55–79. Berkeley: University of
             California Press.

Kanaaneh, Rhoda
2002   Birthing the Nation: Strategies of Palestinian Women in
        Israel. Berkeley: University of California Press.

Karim, Lamia
2008   Demistifying Micro-Credit: The Grameen Bank, NGOs, and
        Neoliberalism in Bangladesh. Cultural Dynamics 20(5):5–30.

Kemper, Robert
1982   The Compadrazago in Urban Mexico. Anthropological Quarterly
        55(1):17–30.

Knaul, Felicia M., Héctor Arreola-Ornelas, Oscar Méndez-Carniado,
Chloe Bryson-Cahn, Jeremy Barofsky, Rachel Maguire, Martha Miranda,
and Sergio Sesma
2007   Las Evidencias Benefician al Sistema de Salud: Reforma para
        Remediar el Gasto Catastrófico y Empobrecedor en Salud en
        México. Salud Pública De México 49(1):70-87.

Kray, Christine A.
2002   The Pentecostal Re-formation of Self: Opting for Orthodoxy in
        Yucatán. Ethos 29(4):395–429.

Kukla, Rebecca
2005   Mass Hysteria: Medicine, Culture and Mothers' Bodies. Lanham:
        Rowman and Littlefield.

Ladd-Taylor, Molly, and Lauri Umansky
1998   Introduction. In "Bad" Mothers: The Politics of Blame in Twentieth-
        Century America. Molly Ladd-Taylor and Lauri Umansky, eds. Pp.
        1–30. New York: New York University Press.

Lamas, Marta
1997   The Feminist Movement and the Development of Political
        Discourse on Voluntary Motherhood in Mexico. Reproductive
        Health Matters 5(10):58–67.

Laveaga, Gabriela S.
2007   "Let's Become Fewer": Soap Operas, Contraception, and
        Nationalizing the Mexican Family in an Overpopulated World.
        Sexuality Research and Social Policy 4(3):19–33.

Lazarus, Ellen
1997   What Do Women Want? Issues of Choice, Control, and Class in
        American Pregnancy and Childbirth. In Childbirth and Authoritative
        Knowledge: Cross-Cultural Perspectives. Robbie E. Davis-Floyd and
        Carolyn F. Sargent, eds. Pp. 132–58. Berkeley: University of California
        Press.

Leatherman, Thomas, and Alan Goodman
2005   Coca-Colonization of Diets in the Yucatan. Social Science and
        Medicine 61(4):833–46.

León-Portilla, Miguel
1962   Obituary: Manuel Gamio, 1883–1960. American Anthropologist
        64(2):356–66.

Lévi-Strauss, Claude
1955   The Structural Study of Myth. Journal of American Folklore
        68(270) 428–44.

Levy, Santiago
2006   Pobreza y Transición Democrática en México: La Continuidad de
        Progresa-Oportunidades. Washington DC: Brookings Institution.

Lindert, Kathy
2006   Brazil: Bolsa Familia Program—Scaling-Up Cash Transfers for the
        Poor. In MfDR Principles in Action: Sourcebook on Emerging Good
        Practices. 67–74. The World Bank. *www.mfdr.org/Sourcebook/1stEdition/*
        MfDRSourcebook-Feb-16-2006.pdf. Accessed August 1, 2012.

Litowitz, Douglas
2000   Gramsci, Hegemony, and the Law. Brigham Young University Law
        Review (2):515–51.

Lock, Margaret
1990   Restoring Order to the House of Japan. Wilson Quarterly
        14(4):42–49.
1993   Cultivating the Body: Anthropology and Epistemologies of
        Bodily Practice and Knowledge. Annual Review of Anthropology
        22:133–55.

Lock, Margaret, and Nancy Scheper-Hughes
1987   The Mindful Body: A Prolegomenon to Future Work in Medical
        Anthropology. Medical Anthropology Quarterly 1(1):6–41.

Lomnitz-Adler, Claudio
1992   Exits from the Labyrinth: Culture and Ideology in the Mexican
        National Space. Berkeley: University of California Press.

Lorenz, Konrad
1974   On Aggression. New York: Harcourt Brace Jovanovich.

MacDonald, Margaret
2006   Gender Expectations: Natural Bodies and Natural Births in the
        New Midwifery in Canada. Medical Anthropology Quarterly
        20(2):235–56.

Mahmood, Cynthia
  1993   Development or Destruction: Walking the Fine Line in Action
         Anthropology. South Asian Monitor, February.

Manderson, Lenore
  1998   Shaping Reproduction: Maternity in Early Twentieth Century
         Malaya. *In* Maternities and Modernities: Colonial and Postcolonial
         Experiences in Asia and the Pacific. Kalpana Ram and Margaret Jolly,
         eds. Pp. 26–50. Cambridge: Cambridge University Press.

Maraesa, Aminata
  2012   A Competition over Reproductive Authority: Prenatal Risk
         Assessment in Southern Belize. *In* Risk, Reproduction, and
         Narratives of Experience. Lauren Fordyce and Aminata Maraesa,
         eds. Pp. 211–29. Nashville: Vanderbilt University Press.

Marentes, Luis A.
  2000   José Vasconcelos and the Writing of the Mexican Revolution. New
         York: Twayne.

Maternowska, M. Catherine
  2006   Reproducing Inequities: Poverty and the Politics of Population in
         Haiti. New Brunswick: Rutgers University Press.

Mauldon, Jane G.
  2003   Providing Subsidies and Incentives for Norplant, Sterilization, and
         Other Contraception: Allowing Economic Theory to Inform Ethical
         Analysis. Journal of Law, Medicine, and Ethics 31:351–64.

Mauss, Marcel
  1973   Techniques of the Body. Economy and Society 2(1):70–88.

Medina, Andrés
  1996   Recuentos y Figuraciones: Ensayos de Antropología
         Mexicana. México, DF: UNAM.

Medlin, Carol, and Damien de Walque
  2008   Potential Applications of Conditional Cash Transfers for Prevention
         of Sexually Transmitted Infections and HIV in Sub-Saharan Africa.
         Policy Research Working Paper 4673. Washington DC: World
         Bank.

México Desconocido
  2011   La Huasteca Potosina: Fascinante por Naturaleza. *www.mexico-
         desconocido.com.mx/la-huasteca-potosina-fascinante-por-naturaleza.html*.
         Accessed February 9, 2011.

Millen, Joyce V., Alec Irwin, and Jim Y. Kim
  2000   Conclusion: Pessimism of the Intellect, Optimism of the Will. *In*
         Dying for Growth: Global Inequality and the Health of the Poor.

Jim Y. Kim, Joyce V. Millen, Alec Irwin, and John Gershman, eds. Pp. 382–90. Monroe, ME: Common Courage.

Miller, Amy C., and Thomas E. Shriver
2012   Women's Childbirth Preferences and Practices in the United States. Social Science and Medicine 75:709–16.

Mitchell, Lisa M.
2006   Body and Illness: Considering Visayan Filipino Children's Perspectives within Local and Global Relationships of Inequality. Medical Anthropology 25:331–73.

Molyneux, Maxine
2000   Twentieth-Century State Formations in Latin America. In Hidden Histories of Gender and the State in Latin America. Elizabeth Dore and Maxine Molyneux, eds. Pp. 33–84. Durham: Duke University Press.
2006   Mothers at the Service of the New Poverty Agenda: Progresa/ Oportunidades, Mexico's Conditional Transfer Programme. Social Policy and Administration 40(4):425–49.
2007   Two Cheers for Conditional Cash Transfers. Institute of Development Studies Bulletin 38(3):69–75.

Montejo, Victor D.
2005   Maya Intellectual Renaissance: Identity, Representation, and Leadership. Austin: University of Texas Press.

Montoya Briones, José J.
1990   Los de Arriba Contra los de Abajo: Testimonios del Terror Caciquil en la Huasteca (1936–1941). In La Huasteca: Vida y Milagros. Cuadernos de la Casa Chata 173. Ludka de Gortari Krauss and Jesús Ruvalcaba Mercado, eds. Pp. 135–56. México, DF: CIESAS-SEP.

Nadal-Melsió, Sara
1996   Dancing Icons or the Syncopation of the Unsayable: Graham's Lamentation and the Cult of the Mater Dolorosa. Lectora: Revista de Dones 2:83–91.

Narayan, Kirin
1993   How Native Is a "Native" Anthropologist? American Anthropologist, New Series 95(3):671–86.

Nava Vite, Rafael
1996   La Huasteca, Uextekapan: Los Pueblos Nahuas en Su Lucha por la Tierra. México, DF: Consejo Nacional para la Cultura y las Artes, Culturas Populares.

2009   El Costumbre: Ofrendas y Música a Chikomexochitl en Ixhuatlán
        de Madero, Veracruz. In Parcela Digital: Comunicación y Desarrollo
        Cultural. Raymundo Aguilera Córdova, ed. Pp. 141–67. Xalapa:
        Universidad Veracruzana Intercultural.

Nazar Beutelspacher, Austreberta, Emma Zapata-Martelo,
and Veronica Vázquez-García
2003   Does Contraception Benefit Women? Structure, Agency, and Well-
        Being in Rural Mexico. Feminist Economics 9(2–3):213–38.

Nigenda, Gustavo, and Maria González-Robledo
2005   Lessons Offered by Latin America's Cash Transfer Programs. Report.
        Mexican Health Foundation, Centre for Social and Economic
        Analysis. London: DFID Health Systems Resource Centre.

Nolasco, Margarita
2003   Medio Siglo de Indigenismo y de INI. Revista México Indígena
        4:32–39.

Oka, Rahul
2008   Resilience and Adaptation of Trade Networks in East African and
        South Asian Port Polities, 1500–1800 C.E. Ph.D. dissertation,
        Department of Anthropology, University of Illinois at Chicago and
        Field Museum of Natural History.

Oka, Rahul, and Agustin Fuentes
2010   From Reciprocity to Trade: How Cooperative Infrastructures Form
        the Basis of Human Socioeconomic Evolution. In Cooperation in
        Social and Economic Life. R. C. Marshal, ed. Pp. 3–28. Walnut
        Creek, CA: Altamira.

Olson, David R., and Nancy Torrance
2001   Conceptualizing Literacy as a Personal Skill and as a Social
        Practice. In The Making of Literate Societies. David R. Olson and
        Nancy Torrance, eds. Pp. 3–18. Oxford: Blackwell.

Ordorica Mellado, Manuel
2006   La Demografía en los Primeros Años del Siglo XXI: Una Visión
        Hacia el Proceso de Envejecimiento. Papeles de Población 50:23-35.

Ortiz-Ortega, Adriana, and Mercedes Barquet
2010   Gendering Transition to Democracy in Mexico. Latin American
        Research Review 45:108–37.

Overmyer-Velázquez, Rebecca
2003   The Self-Determination of Indigenous Peoples and the Limits
        of United Nations Advocacy in Guerrero, Mexico (1998–2000).
        Identities: Global Studies in Culture and Power 10:9–29.

Pender, John
2001   From "Structural Adjustment" to "Comprehensive Development
        Framework": Conditionality Transformed? Third World Quarterly
        22(3):397–411.

Pérez Zevallos, Juan M.
1998   Las Visitas de la Huasteca (Siglos XVI–XVIII). *In* Nuevos Aportes
        al Conocimiento de la Huasteca. J. Ruvalcaba Mercado, ed. Pp.
        95–122. México, DF: CIESAS; Centro de Investigaciones Históricas
        de San Luis Potosí; CEMCA; INI.

Petchesky, Rosalind P.
1995   From Population Control to Reproductive Rights: Feminist Fault
        Lines. Reproductive Health Matters 3(6):152–61.

Pigg, Stacy Leigh
1997   Authority in Translation: Finding, Knowing, Naming, and
        Training "Traditional Birth Attendants" in Nepal. *In* Childbirth
        and Authoritative Knowledge: Cross-Cultural Perspectives. Robbie
        Davis-Floyd and Carolyn F. Sargent, eds. Pp. 233–62. Berkeley:
        University of California Press.

Pilcher, Jeffrey
2000   El Signo de la Mugre: Cantinflas, Cross-Dressing, and the Creation
        of a Mexican Mass Audience. Journal of Latin American Cultural
        Studies 9(3):333–48.

Provost, Jean-Paul
2004   El Carnaval en la Huasteca Indígena: Un Análisis de Su Significado
        Funcional. *In* La Huasteca, un Recorrido por Su Diversidad. Jesús
        Ruvalcaba Mercado, Juan Manuel Pérez Zevallos, and Octavio
        Herrera Pérez, eds. Pp. 267–94. México, DF: CIESAS.

Public Radio International
2009   Mexico's Anti-poverty Program, Oportunidades. *www.pri.org/stories/
        business/Global-Development/mexico-anti-povery-program.html*.
        Accessed December 31, 2011.

Purcell, Trevor
1998   Indigenous Knowledge and Applied Anthropology: Questions of
        Definition and Direction. Human Organization 57(3):258–72.

Pylypa, Jen
1998   Power and Bodily Practice: Applying the Work of Foucault to an
        Anthropology of the Body. Arizona Anthropologist 13:21–36.

Radcliffe-Browne, Alfred
1940   On Joking Relationships. Africa: Journal of the International African
        Institute 13(3):195–210.

Ram, Kalpana, and Margaret Jolly
  1998   Maternities and Modernities: Colonial and Postcolonial Experiences
          in Asia and the Pacific. Cambridge: Cambridge University Press.

Razavi, Shahra, and Carol Miller
  1995   From WID to GAD: Conceptual Shifts in the Women and
          Development Discourse. Occasional Paper 1, February 1995. United
          Nations Research Institute for Social Development. United Nations
          Development Programme.

Reeves, Hazel, and Sally Baden
  2000   Gender and Development: Concepts and Definitions. Report No.
          55. Institute of Development Studies, University of Sussex.

Rivera, Juan A., Daniel Sotres-Alvarez, Daniel Habicht, Teresa Shamah,
and Salvador Villalpando
  2004   Impact of the Mexican Program of Education, Health, and
          Nutrition (Progresa) on Rates of Growth and Anemia in Infants and
          Young Children: A Randomized Effectiveness Study. Journal of the
          American Medical Association 291(21):2563–70.

Robertson, Jennifer
  2002   Reflexivity Redux: A Pithy Polemic on "Positionality."
          Anthropological Quarterly 75(4):785–92.

Robinson, Vera
  1970   Humor in Nursing. American Journal of Nursing 70(5):1065–69.

Rosenbaum, Rainer
  1995   Mexico Creates New Directorate of Reproductive Health. United
          Nations Population Information Network. *www.un.org/popin/
          unfpa/taskforce/icpdnews/icpdnews9507/mexico.asc.html.* Accessed
          April 13, 2011.

Ruhl, Lealle
  2002   Dilemmas of the Will: Uncertainty, Reproduction, and the Rhetoric
          of Control. Signs 27(3):641–63.

Ruvalcaba Mercado, Jesús
  1998a   Notas Sobre las Plantas Cultivadas y los Animales Domésticos de la
          Huasteca. *In* Nuevos Aportes al Conocimiento de la Huasteca. Jesús
          Ruvalcaba Mercado, ed. Pp. 39–57. México, DF: CIESAS.
  1998b   Presentación. *In* Nuevos Aportes al Conocimiento de la Huasteca.
          Jesús Mercado Ruvalcaba, ed. Pp. 11–29. México, DF: CIESAS.
  2004   La Agricultura de Roza en la Huasteca, ¿Suicido o Tesoro Colectivo?
          In La Huasteca, un Recorrido por Su Diversidad. Jesús Ruvalcaba
          Mercado, Juan Manuel Pérez Zevallos, and Octavio Herrera Pérez,
          eds. México, DF: CIESAS.

Ruvalcaba Mercado, Jesús, Juan Manuel Pérez Zevallos, and Octavio Herrera
2004   Presentación. *In* La Huasteca, un Recorrido por Su Diversidad.
        Jesús Ruvalcaba Mercado, Juan Manuel Pérez Zevallos, and Octavio
        Herrera, eds. Pp. 11–14. México, DF: CIESAS.

Saith, Ashwani
2006   From Universal Values to Millennium Development Goals: Lost in
        Translation. Development and Change 37(6):1167–99.

Sánchez, Consuelo
1999   Los Pueblos Indígenas: Del Indigenismo a la Autonomía. México,
        DF: Siglo XXI Editores.

Sandstrom, Alan R.
1975   Ecology, Economy, and the Realm of the Sacred: An Interpretation
        of Ritual in a Nahua Community of the Southern Huasteca, Mexico.
        Ph.D. dissertation, Department of Anthropology, Indiana University,
        Bloomington.
1991   Corn Is Our Blood: Culture and Ethnic Identity in a Contemporary
        Aztec Village. Norman: University of Oklahoma Press.
1998   El Nene Lloroso y el Espíritu Nahua del Maíz: El Cuerpo Humano
        como Símbolo Clave en la Huasteca Veracruzana. *In* Nuevos Aportes
        al Conocimiento de la Huasteca. Jesús Ruvalcaba Mercado, ed. Pp.
        59–94. México, DF: CIESAS.
2003   Nahua Blood Sacrifice and Pilgrimage to Sacred Mountain
        Postectli, June 2001. Report Submitted to the Foundation for
        the Advancement of Mesoamerican Studies. *www.famsi.org/
        reports/01001/01001Sandstrom01.pdf*. Accessed January 26, 2006.

Sandstrom, Alan R., and Arturo Gómez Martínez
2004   Petición a Chicomexochitl: Un Canto al Espíritu del Maíz, por la
        Chamana Nahua Silveria Hernández Hernández. *In* La Huasteca,
        un Recorrido por Su Diversidad. Jesús Ruvalcaba Mercado, Juan
        Manuel Pérez Zevallos, and Octavio Herrera Pérez, eds. Pp. 343–68.
        México, DF: CIESAS.

Sanz Jara, Eva
2009   La Crisis del Indigenismo Clásico y el Surgimiento de un Nuevo
        Paradigma sobre la Población Indígena de México. Revista
        Complutense de Historia de América 35:257–81.

Sargent, Carolyn F.
2005   Counseling Contraception for Malian Migrants in Paris: Global,
        State, and Personal Politics. Human Organization 64(2):147–56.

Sargent, Carolyn F., and Caroline B. Brettell, eds.
1996   Gender and Health: An International Perspective. Upper Saddle
        River: Prentice Hall.

Sawicki, Jana
1999   Disciplining Mothers: Feminism and the New Reproductive
        Technologies. *In* Feminist Theory and the Body: A Reader. Janet
        Price and Margrit Shildrick, eds. Pp. 190–202. London: Routledge.

Sawyer, Suzana, and Arun Agrawal
2000   Environmental Orientalisms. Cultural Critique 45:71–108.

Schedler, Andreas
2004   'El Voto Es Nuestro': Como los Ciudadanos Mexicanos Perciben
        el Clientelismo Electoral. Revista Mexicana de Sociología
        66(1):61–101.

Scheper-Hughes, Nancy
1993   Death without Weeping: The Violence of Everyday Life in Brazil.
        Berkeley: University of California Press.
2002   Disease or Deception: Munchausen by Proxy as a Weapon of the
        Weak. Anthropology and Medicine 9(2):153–73.

Scott, James
1985   Weapons of the Weak: Everyday Forms of Peasant Resistance. New
        Haven: Yale University Press.
1990   Domination and the Arts of Resistance: The Hidden Transcripts of
        Subordinate Groups. New Haven: Yale University Press.
1998   Seeing Like a State: How Certain Schemes to Improve the Human
        Condition Have Failed. New Haven: Yale University Press.

Secretaría de Desarrollo Social (SEDESOL)
2003   Manual Cuidado 2003: SEDESOL a Los Ojos de Todos. México,
        DF: Secretaría de Desarrollo Social, Secretaría de la Función Pública,
        Transparencia Mexicana, FEPADE.
2009   Listado de Localidades y Número de Familias Beneficiarias al Inicio
        del Ejercicio Fiscal 2009, Veracruz. *www.oportunidades.gob.mx/
        Portal/wb/Web/listado_de_localidades_y_numero_de_familias_2009.*
        Accessed August 8, 2012.
2011   Reglas de Operación del Programa de Desarrollo Humano
        Oportunidades 2011. *www.oportunidades.gob.mx/Portal/wb/Web/
        reglas_de_operacion_del_oportunidades_2011.* Accessed August 2,
        2012.
2012a   Manual Cuidado 2012: SEDESOL a Los Ojos de Todos. México,
        DF: Secretaría de Desarrollo Social, Secretaría de la Función Pública,
        Transparencia Mexicana, FEPADE.
2012b   Oportunidades Cumple 15 Años de Incentivar el Desarrollo Humano
        de Quienes Más lo Necesitan. *www.oportunidades.gob.mx/Portal/wb/
        Web/oportunidades_cumple_15_anos_de_incentivar.* Accessed August 2,
        2012.

Secretaría de Salud
    2002   El Derecho a la Libre Decisión en Salud Reproductiva. México, DF:
            Secretaría de Salud.

Sen, Amartya
    1999   Development as Freedom. Oxford: Oxford University Press.

Sesia, Paola
    1996   "Women Come Here on Their Own When They Need To": Prenatal
            Care, Authoritative Knowledge, and Maternal Health in Oaxaca.
            Medical Anthropology Quarterly 10(2):121–40.
    2007   Reproductive Health and Reproductive Rights after the Cairo
            Consensus: Accomplishments and Shortcomings in the Establishment
            of Innovative Public Policies in Oaxaca. Sexuality Research and Social
            Policy:4(3) 34–49.

Sherzer, Joel
    2002   Speech Play and Verbal Art. Austin: University of Texas Press.

Skoufias, Emmanuel
    2005   PROGRESA and Its Impacts on the Welfare of Rural Households in
            Mexico: Research Report 139. Washington, DC: International Food
            Policy Research Institute.

Smith-Oka, Vania
    2008   Plants Used for Reproductive Health by Nahua Women in Northern
            Veracruz, Mexico. Journal of Economic Botany 62(4):604–14.
    2009   Unintended Consequences: Exploring the Tensions between
            Development Programs and Indigenous Women in Mexico in the
            Context of Reproductive Health. Social Science and Medicine
            68:2069–77.
    2012   "They Don't Know Anything": How Medical Authority Constructs
            Perceptions of Reproductive Risk among Low-Income Mothers
            in Mexico. In Risk, Reproduction, and Narratives of Experience.
            Lauren Fordyce and Aminata Maraesa, eds. Pp. 103–21. Nashville:
            Vanderbilt University Press.

Sridhar, Devi, and Arabella Duffield
    2006   A Review of the Impact of Cash Transfer Programmes on Child
            Nutritional Status and Some Implications for Save the Children UK
            Programmes. Report. London: Save the Children, UK.

Stavenhagen, Rodolfo
    1991   The Ethnic Question: Conflicts, Development, and Human Rights.
            Tokyo: United Nations University Press.
    1997   Las Organizaciones Indígenas: Actores Emergentes en América
            Latina. In Identidades Étnicas. Manuel Gutiérrez, ed. Pp. 13–41.
            Madrid: Casa de América.

Stern, Alexandra M.
1999   Responsible Mothers and Normal Children: Eugenics, Nationalism, and Welfare in Post-Revolutionary Mexico, 1920–1940. Journal of Historical Sociology 12(4):369–97.

Szeljak, György
2003   ". . . Porque Si No Comemos Maíz No Vivimos." Identidad y Ritos de Fertilidad en la Huasteca Hidalguense. *In* ¡Viva la Huasteca! Jóvenes Miradas sobre la Región. Juan Manuel Pérez Zevallos and Jesús Ruvalcaba Mercado, eds. Pp. 113–44. México, DF: CIESAS.

Tapias, Maria
2006   Emotions and the Intergenerational Embodiment of Social Suffering in Rural Bolivia. Medical Anthropology Quarterly 20(3):399–415.

Thornton, Rebecca
2003   The Demand for, and Impact of, Learning HIV Status. American Economics Review 98(5):1829–63.

Tsing, Anna L.
1990   Monster Stories: Women Charged with Prenatal Endangerment. *In* Uncertain Terms: Negotiating Gender in American Culture. Faye Ginsburg and Anna L. Tsing, eds. Pp. 282–99. Boston: Beacon.

Tuirán, Rodolfo, Virgilio Partida, Octavio Mojarro, and Elena Zúñiga
2002   Tendencias y Perspectivas de la Fecundidad. *In* La Situación Demográfica de México, 2002. Pp. 29–48. México, DF: Consejo Nacional de Población.

United Nations (UN)
2011   Outcomes on Gender and Equality. *www.un.org/en/development/ devagenda/gender.shtml*. Accessed December 15, 2011.

Van Hollen, Cecilia
2003   Birth on the Threshold: Childbirth and Modernity in South India. Berkeley: University of California Press.

van Hooft, Anuschka
2007   The Ways of the Water: A Reconstruction of Huastecan Nahua Society through its Oral Tradition. Amsterdam: Amsterdam University Press.

Vasconcelos, José
1925   La Raza Cósmica. Madrid: Agencia Mundial de Librería.

Vaughn, Mary Kay
2000   Modernizing Patriarchy: State Policies, Rural Households, and Women in Mexico, 1930–1940. *In* Hidden Histories of Gender and the State in Latin America. Elizabeth Dore and Maxine Molyneux, eds. Pp. 194–214. Durham: Duke University Press.

Viveros-Añorve, José
    2012   The Opportunity Cost of Financing Progresa-Oportunidades.
            Research Proposal, Center for Development Research, University of
            Bonn.

Warman, Arturo
    1970   Presentación: Todos Santos y Todos Difuntos. *In* De Eso Que Llaman
            Antropología Mexicana. Arturo Warman, ed. Pp. 7–38. México, DF:
            Editorial Nuestro Tiempo.

Wetterberg, Anna
    2004   My Body, My Choice . . . My Responsibility: The Pregnant Woman
            as Caretaker of the Fetal Person. Berkeley Journal of Sociology
            48:27–48.

Whiteford, Linda M.
    1996   Political Economy, Gender, and the Social Production of Health
            and Illness. *In* Gender and Health: An International Perspective.
            Carolyn F. Sargent and Caroline B. Brettell, eds. Pp. 242–59.
            Upper Saddle River: Prentice-Hall.
    2000   Local Identity, Globalization, and Health in Cuba and the
            Dominican Republic. *In* Global Health Policy, Local Realities: The
            Fallacy of the Level Playing Field. Linda M. Whiteford and Lenore
            Manderson, eds. Pp. 57–78. Boulder: Lynne Rienner.

Whiteford, Linda M., and Lenore Manderson
    2000   Introduction: Health, Globalization, and the Fallacy of the Level
            Playing Field. *In* Global Health Policy, Local Realities: The Fallacy
            of the Level Playing Field. Linda M. Whiteford and Lenore
            Manderson, eds. Pp. 1–19. Boulder: Lynne Rienner.

White House
    2001   National Family Week Proclamation. November 21, 2001.
            georgewbush-whitehouse.archives.gov/news/releases/2001/11/
            20011121-1.html. Accessed August 3, 2012.

Whyte, Susan R., Sjaak van der Geest, and Anita Hardon
    2002   Social Lives of Medicine. Cambridge: Cambridge University Press.

Wilk, Richard
    2011   Poverty and Excess in a Binge Economy. Paper presented at the
            Annual Meeting of the Society for Economic Anthropology, Notre
            Dame, IN, March 11, 2011.

Wodon, Quentin, Benedicte de la Briere, Corinne Siaens, and Shlomo Yitzhaki
    2003   Mexico's PROGRESA: Innovative Targeting, Gender Focus and
            Impact on Social Welfare. En Breve 17:1–4.

World Health Organization (WHO)
    2008   Skilled Birth Attendants. World Health Organization. *www.who.int/maternal_child_adolescent/topics/maternal/skilled_birth/en/index.html.* Accessed October 3, 2011.

Yoels, William C., and Jeffery M. Clair
    1995   Laughter in the Clinic: Humor as Social Organization. Symbolic Interaction 18(1):39–58.

Index